More praise for *The Interstitial Cystitis Solution*:

" . . . presents an organized, step-by-step, holistic approach to treating IC and empowers the patient . . .
a 'must read' for those dealing with IC. Nicole is truly an authority in the area of interstitial cystitis!"
—Barb Zarnikow, board co-chair, Interstitial Cystitis Association,
IC patient, support group leader, and patient advocate

"*The Interstitial Cystitis Solution* is a godsend for those dealing with the diagnosis of IC. A recognized leader in the
treatment of IC, Dr. Nicole Cozean has masterfully blended her knowledge and clinical expertise to provide the
reader with a user-friendly guide to help navigate the many challenges associated with this diagnosis."
—Steve Ferdig, P.T., D.P.T., O.C.S., C.N.P., adjunct clinical faculty, Chapman University,
and owner, Specialized Physical Therapy

" . . . thorough, readable, and masterfully well-organized. Cozean offers helpful reviews, takeaways, myth alerts,
as well as charts and templates for recordkeeping. The book is most helpful in passing on this expert's
knowledge to patients who wish to more successfully manage the condition. I highly recommend
The Interstitial Cystitis Solution for all patients with IC and their caregivers, both personal and professional."
—Joy Selak, board member, Interstitial Cystitis Association,
and coauthor, *You Don't Look Sick! Living Well with Invisible Chronic Illness*

"Nicole presents the most crucial information about IC/PBS in a thorough yet easy-to-read format
and helps readers use this information to develop their unique plan for healing.
This book is a guidebook for the healing journey, and Nicole is the ultimate guide."
—Mary Ruth Velicki, P.T., D.P.T., M.S.P.T., author of *Healing through Chronic Pain*

" . . . packed with up-to-date and valuable information to help empower both patients and clinicians alike.
This book provides education, support, and resources for those struggling with this often misdiagnosed
and painful condition. This comprehensive guide will provide you with the tools necessary to support
you along your healing journey. You can get your life back, and this book will show you how."
—Laura Ricci, P.T., D.P.T., W.H.N.C., certified women's health and nutrition coach

For my patients

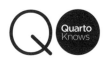

Quarto is the authority on a wide range of topics.

Quarto educates, entertains and enriches the lives of our readers—enthusiasts and lovers of hands-on living.

www.QuartoKnows.com

Text © 2016 Nicole Cozean, P.T., D.P.T, W.C.S., and Jesse Cozean

First published in the United States of America in 2016 by
Fair Winds Press, an imprint of
Quarto Publishing Group USA Inc.
100 Cummings Center
Suite 406-L
Beverly, Massachusetts 01915-6101
Telephone: (978) 282-9590
Fax: (978) 283-2742
QuartoKnows.com
Visit our blogs at QuartoKnows.com

20 19 18 17 16   1 2 3 4 5

ISBN: 978-1-59233-737-8

Digital edition published in 2016.

Library of Congress Cataloging-in-Publication Data

Names: Cozean, Nicole, author. | Cozean, Jesse.
Title: The interstitial cystitis solution : a holistic plan for healing painful symptoms, resolving bladder and pelvic floor dysfunction, and taking back your life / Nicole Cozean, D.P.T., P.T., W.C.S., C.S.C.S., and Jesse Cozean.
Description: Beverly, Massachusetts : Fair Winds Press, 2016.
Identifiers: LCCN 2016022966| ISBN 9781592337378 (paperback) | ISBN 9781631592089 (eisbn)
Subjects: LCSH: Interstitial cystitis--Popular works. | Interstitial cystitis--Alternative treatment--Popular works. | Bladder--Diseases--Diet therapy--Popular works. | BISAC: HEALTH & FITNESS / Diseases / Genitourinary & STDs. | HEALTH & FITNESS / Diseases / General. | HEALTH & FITNESS / Women's Health.
Classification: LCC RC921.C9 C69 2016 | DDC 616.6/23--dc23
LC record available at https://lccn.loc.gov/2016022966

Cover and book design: Kathie Alexander
Photography: Brad Herman
Fitness model: Rebecca Beckler
Illustrations: Mattie Wells

Printed in China

The information in this book is for educational purposes only. It is not intended to replace the advice of a physician or medical practitioner. Please see your health-care provider before beginning any new health program.

THE
INTERSTITIAL
CYSTITIS
SOLUTION

A Holistic Plan for Healing Painful Symptoms, Resolving Bladder and Pelvic Floor Dysfunction, and Taking Back Your Life

**NICOLE COZEAN, P.T., D.P.T., W.C.S.,
AND
JESSE COZEAN**

FAIR WINDS

CONTENTS

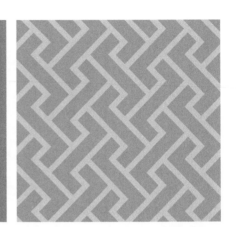

INTRODUCTION

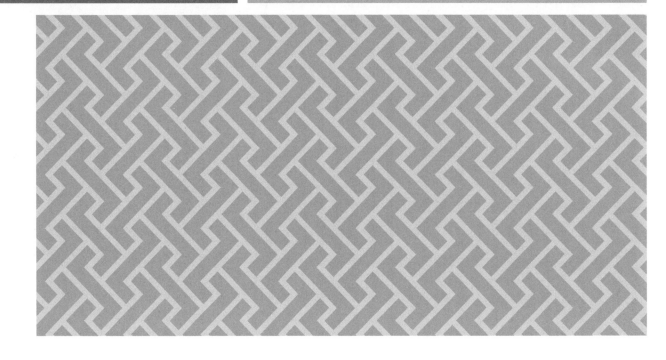

Thousands of people with interstitial cystitis (IC) live healthy, pain-free lives, and so can you. I'm writing this book to share that message with patients far beyond the walls of my own clinic.

As a physical therapist, I help patients every day who struggle with the pain and urinary symptoms of IC. I see my patients several times a week and get involved in their lives. I'm on the front lines, learning what works and what doesn't—sharing in the frustration when a flare compromises valuable progress or the joy of being able to return to work or go on a family vacation for the first time in years. Yes, interstitial cystitis is a difficult condition to manage, but there is hope. With dedicated effort, you can regain control of your health.

My patients are the inspiration behind this book. Many of them struggled with IC for years, shuttling from doctor to doctor before being diagnosed. Worse, some were quickly dismissed by their doctors, told the pain was all in their heads. And even after being diagnosed, many of my patients found little relief with the constant barrage of prescriptions and procedures and weren't even given the most basic information about the condition. That's why teaching my patients about the condition and how they can affect it is almost as important as the physical therapy we do.

Healing interstitial cystitis symptoms is a journey. It requires a holistic approach and a combination of treatments and therapies. Simply put, you *can* get your life back.

Information Overload

Once upon a time, there wasn't enough information available about interstitial cystitis. Now, there's almost too much. Well-meaning patients share stories of this wonder drug or that miracle procedure on Internet forums or Facebook pages. Someone suffering a flare may blame a specific food, medication, or activity. Drug companies and the manufacturers of dietary supplements promote their own products, while researchers constantly propose new theories that other researchers test and disprove. All of this can be overwhelming, contradictory, and confusing.

Are You Overwhelmed or Hyperfocused?

I've noticed the majority of my patients fall into one of two categories after an interstitial cystitis diagnosis. Recognizing which tendency you have is important because either can become a roadblock to recovery.

Some people are overwhelmed by the condition and all the information available on it. Many haven't received a good description of the condition from their doctors and don't understand what the diagnosis means! With so much uncertainty, it can be difficult to know where to start. If this sounds familiar, take heart: This book provides practical advice you can begin to follow immediately to improve your symptoms and regain control of your life.

Others have the opposite reaction when they receive their diagnosis. Instead of being overwhelmed, they find something specific and tangible to focus on. The object of this focus can vary widely. It might be a particular symptom or a specific phrase used by a doctor. Some patients have strong feelings about what caused their condition or what the best treatment option is. These patients are easy to spot. They walk in the door with overflowing stacks of paper in their arms, each article covered in highlighter or filled with notes. If you fall into this category, the challenge is broadening your viewpoint to include new information that may not fit neatly into your original theories. Ultimately, there is no simple answer to the problem of interstitial cystitis; healing requires a multidisciplinary approach.

These different tendencies can prevent you from acting to manage your condition. If you struggle with feeling overwhelmed, find something practical to do that helps your symptoms. If you tend to focus on one particular aspect of the condition, challenge yourself to try something new, even if you're skeptical about it. Don't become paralyzed by your preconceptions.

Managing Your IC

As you begin to manage your IC, keep these three things in mind:

1. **There is hope.** I've worked with IC and pelvic pain patients for more than ten years. With appropriate treatment, physical therapy, exercises, and lifestyle changes, everyone can achieve substantial reductions in pain and urinary symptoms. For many people, symptoms disappear almost entirely and they learn to handle the occasional flare when it occurs.

2. **There are no easy answers.** There's no miracle pill that works for everyone with IC, nor is there a medical procedure that guarantees relief. And there hasn't been a new, FDA-approved medication for IC since 1996. All this means that you'll undergo some trial and error as you discover what works for you and your body. It will require a holistic approach—

a combination of treatments that work together to relieve pain and urinary symptoms. Most importantly, it takes perseverance to push through frustrations and setbacks.

3. **Take control of your health.** No one you meet will care as much about your health as you do. You'll need to do your own research, keep track of your symptoms, and learn what does and doesn't work with your condition. Finding a good medical team is essential, but you can't depend entirely on your doctor or physical therapist. With IC, there are some things out of your control— and that means you have to control whatever you can. Diet, exercise, stretching, posture, and stress management can all result in major, sustainable improvements in your symptoms.

Your IC Journey: A New Path

Whether you've just been diagnosed with IC or only suspect you have interstitial cystitis but have not received a formal diagnosis from a doctor, this can also be an overwhelming time. Many patients feel a sense of relief, though, when they're finally able to give a name to their condition. And it's encouraging to know many people are able to manage their symptoms successfully and return to their normal lives.

However, there's no single pill or procedure that's universally effective, and almost all IC medications are actually drugs originally created for other conditions. The treatments prescribed by doctors can vary widely: You'll hear about oral medications, medicine inserted directly into the bladder, physical therapy, and, perhaps, nontraditional remedies, such as acupuncture. The elimination diet will make its way into your vocabulary. You'll learn that what you eat can influence symptoms, and you'll start to adjust your eating habits. Lifestyle changes will be necessary, as well. You may find it difficult to sit in a car or at a desk for long periods of time, and the location of the nearest bathroom becomes vital knowledge. Periods of stress tend to cause symptom flares. Stretching may become an important part of your daily routine.

It's true that IC is a condition that manifests differently in each person. This book will help you navigate your path with practical, positive information, guiding you to make the best decisions and prioritize treatment options as you take control of your health. You're going on a lifelong trek. Sure, you'll trip over rocks and skin your knees along the way. But there'll also be long, smooth downhill stretches that will make it all worthwhile. For now, though, the most important thing is to lace up your boots and take your first step.

Your IC Journey: A Well-Worn Path

At the other end of the spectrum are people who have wrestled with this condition for years. If you're one of those people, dietary restrictions and different medications will be old news to you. You may have your symptoms mostly under control, with only the occasional flare. Or you might still be struggling, your stumped doctors still searching for the medication or treatment that will finally help. You may be exhausted at the thought of making yet another change to your lifestyle, or of trying yet another strategy. This book can help.

Think of it this way: You've been on this journey for a while. There are holes in your boots and your backpack feels heavier. For you, the first thing to do is to set that backpack down for a while. Unpack it. Take a look at everything you're carrying with you. Is it helping you—or is it just dead weight that you can leave behind?

You're coming to this book with a lot of hard-won information about your condition and your body. That information is invaluable, and this book will ask you to apply your knowledge to guide you to success. I'll also ask you to keep an open mind and reevaluate some of your long-held ideas. Research on IC is accelerating, and we know substantially more about it now than we did even a few years ago. No matter how long you've had the condition, I can promise you'll learn something new and helpful from this book.

What's Unique About This Book?

Much of the information you'll find on IC promotes only a certain philosophy of treatment. Doctors tend to focus exclusively on the bladder, and prescribe bladder and generalized pain medications that only mask symptoms. Physical therapists deal with the musculoskeletal causes of pain, but can't offer prescription medications. Nutritionists can work with your diet, but have nothing to say about the bladder or pelvic floor. Other practitioners focus on alternative medicine, acupuncture, meditation, or dietary supplements.

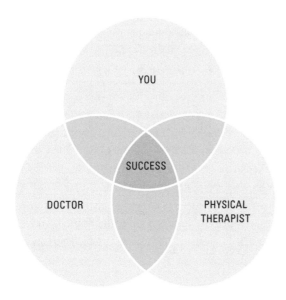

This book is different. Healing really does take a multidisciplinary approach, and it's the result of the combined efforts of you and your medical team. Your doctor can help with medications; your physical therapist (PT) can help with your pelvic floor; but only you can take the necessary steps that bring about true recovery—alterations to your diet, self-care, and the mental approach. Everyone is different, and there are many paths to healing: We hope the positive, practical information in this book helps you find yours.

How to Use This Book

This book is divided into three sections. Section I provides an overview of interstitial cystitis and gives you background information and current research to help you understand this complicated condition. Section II focuses on the different treatment options. More than 180 different treatments have been proposed and tested, and this section summarizes the research, including the options with the highest probability of success. It also discusses traditional medications, physical therapy, diet and lifestyle changes, and alternative medicine. Section III is your roadmap—a step-by-step program for developing a unique, holistic combination of treatments that work for you.

ho·lis·tic (adjective)
Characterized by the treatment of the whole person … rather than just the physical symptoms of a disease.

The best maps are tattered and torn by the end of the journey. So go ahead and highlight sections here that are important to you. Make notes about treatments that worked and those that didn't. Put asterisks or stars next to helpful advice and draw angry faces next to things that don't work for you. (If you're reading this as an eBook, keep a notebook handy to jot down your thoughts as you read.) This is a resource for you; use it in whichever way is most helpful.

This book also includes questionnaires and surveys to help you evaluate your symptoms and give you valuable information about the condition. Some are meant to be used only once, but others are designed to track your symptoms over time. Feel free to copy them out of the book, re-create them yourself, or visit us at PelvicSanity.com for printable versions.

I do my best to avoid medical terminology and jargon whenever possible. So if I do use a technical term, there's a reason; it's important for you to be familiar with it.

The end of each chapter features a section on the major take-away points. These summarize what you've learned and can refresh your memory as you flip back through the book after you're finished.

You Are Not a Statistic

Remember, you're a person, not a statistic. Even if a treatment works 95 percent of the time, some people won't gain any benefit from it. And that also means not everything you read in this book will help you. Yes, it walks you through the common treatments for IC and the likelihood of success, but it's up to you to gauge how your body responds. There is no right or wrong way to treat IC—only ways that work and ways that don't. So, if it works for you, keep it; if it doesn't, discard it. Are you ready to start?

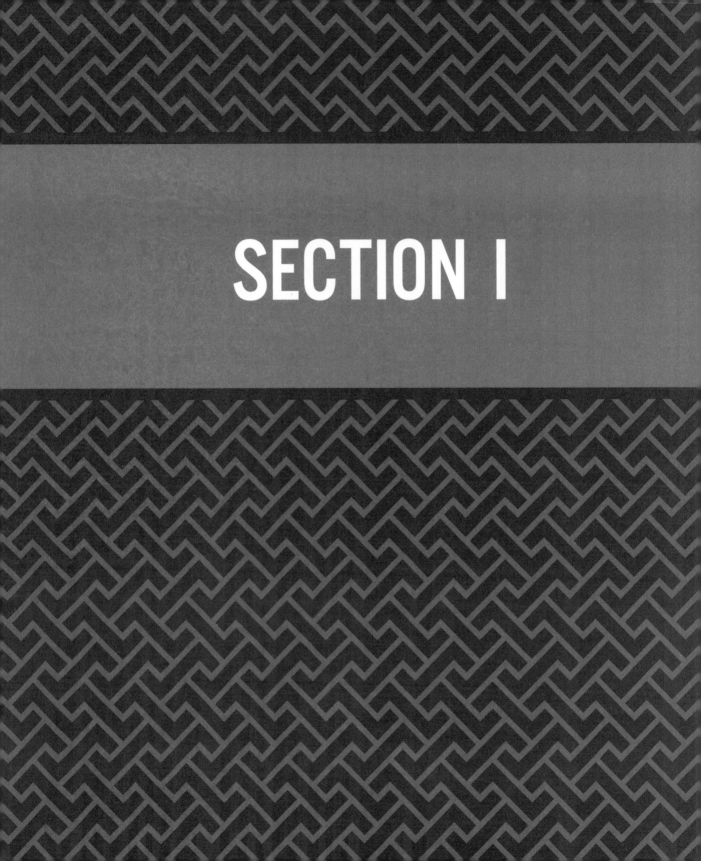

SECTION I

Interstitial Cystitis (IC) Overview

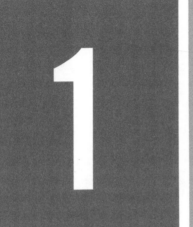

The Big Picture:

An Overview of IC

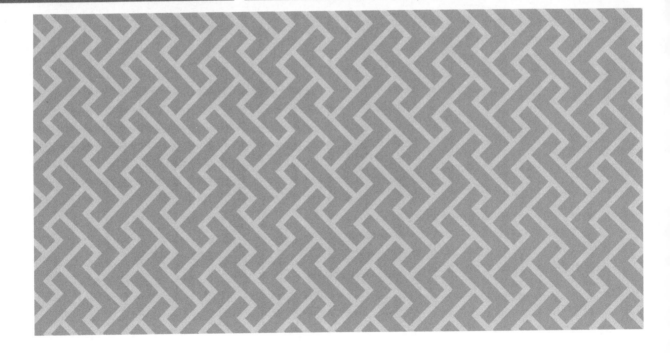

F inding an accepted definition of interstitial cystitis is a challenge. Experts have argued over the exact language and terminology for IC for almost 150 years, which means there's still a lot of confusion for patients and practitioners.

What Is IC?

IC is a chronic pain and bladder condition that typically causes both pelvic pain and urinary symptoms, including increased frequency and an urgent need to use the bathroom. It can be diagnosed once symptoms are present for more than six weeks, and in the absence of any other condition that would offer an explanation, such as a urinary tract infection. The simplest definition of IC, then, is discomfort or pain that feels related to the bladder and is accompanied by urinary symptoms without any other known cause.

"Cystitis" is the medical term for inflammation of the bladder. The word "interstitial" is less specific, and refers to an in-between space—in this case, the lining of the bladder. The condition is chronic, meaning it is long lasting, but is not degenerative: That is, there is no intrinsic reason for symptoms to get worse over time, and they can certainly improve with proper treatment.

History of IC

First recognized by the medical community in the early 1800s, IC was initially categorized as a bladder tic, suggesting a nerve problem as the root of the condition. The term "interstitial cystitis" was coined in 1876, and the name reflects the impact of inflammation in the bladder. Today, it's understood that both inflammation and the nervous system play major roles in IC.

In 1914, around the start of World War I, a urologist named Guy LeRoy Hunner found "elusive ulcers" in the bladders of some patients with the condition, and these ulcers now bear his name (Hunner's lesions). These wounds in the bladder lining dominated the scientific approach to IC for more than fifty years. Researchers assumed all IC patients either had lesions or would inevitably develop them. A vocal portion of the medical community believed IC wasn't a real condition at all, because many people who reported symptoms didn't have these bladder ulcerations. It wasn't until 1978 that Stanford researchers demonstrated the vast majority of patients with IC do not have Hunner's lesions, proving the condition could not be defined by these wounds in the bladder wall.

The Stigma of IC

Because many patients—almost exclusively women—complained of pain without an obvious physical explanation, many doctors concluded their symptoms were "in their head" (psychosomatic) and dismissed the symptoms as products of female hysteria. This stigma has persisted throughout the history of the condition, and still affects how it is perceived, diagnosed, and treated today.

IC in the 1970s

"A medical entity [IC] as confusing, poorly understood, baffling etiologically, and taking up as much space as it does in the textbooks on urology should merit a few words from a psychiatrist . . . it makes a thoughtful physician wonder about the possibility of a mildly masochistic woman, i.e., destructive need in the female, to suffer and to 'have trouble with' her genitourinary apparatus." *Urology,* vol. 3, Meredith F. Campbell, ed. (1970).

Through the 1970s, doctors were taught that interstitial cystitis was a physical manifestation of masochistic, emotionally unbalanced, and disturbed women. This attitude permeated the medical community, and was passed on to younger doctors as they progressed through medical school. A formal definition of interstitial cystitis wasn't created until 1987, and the American Urological Association finally published their first guideline on IC in 2011. It is no wonder, then, that many practitioners may be equipped with out-of-date information about interstitial cystitis, and so the stigma associated with the condition continues. Too many of my patients are told to "drink some cranberry juice" or "relax and have a glass of wine" when they report their excruciating pain to their doctors. With the challenges inherent in diagnosing and treating interstitial cystitis, concocting a simpler explanation, such as psychological problems, can be tempting.

Though it's unfair that these stigmas still exist, they're part of the reality you'll face as you travel on your IC journey. Throughout this book, I'll offer advice about the best way to interact with your doctor and the wider medical community. How you present yourself and your condition when you first see a new doctor is extremely important. That said, I don't mean to suggest all medical practitioners are behind the times. There are some fantastic specialists who work very hard to stay current with new research. If you find one, he or she can be an invaluable resource.

Names for IC

Interstitial cystitis has been given various names over the years, causing confusion for patients and practitioners alike. Following is a brief summary of some other names and their origins so you'll recognize them if you see them in other sources; throughout this book, however, I only refer to the condition as "interstitial cystitis."

Seeking a name that better described the condition, researchers proposed Painful Bladder Syndrome (PBS) in the early 2000s. They wanted to separate the term from interstitial cystitis, which would only be used for "classic" IC patients with Hunner's lesions. Unfortunately, they failed to describe the differences between the conditions adequately, so the two terms became synonymous and eventually merged into IC/PBS.

Alphabet Soup: Alternative Terms for Interstitial Cystitis

IC Interstitial Cystitis
BPS Bladder Pain Syndrome
HBS Hypersensitive Bladder Syndrome
HSB Hypersensitive Bladder
PBS Painful Bladder Syndrome
IC/PBS Interstitial Cystitis/Painful Bladder Syndrome
UCPPS Urologic Chronic Pelvic Pain Syndrome

What Causes IC?

Unfortunately, little is known about the underlying cause(s) of interstitial cystitis. Researchers have proposed many theories but with little supporting evidence. In all likelihood, IC is the result of a complex combination of factors, not a single cause.

Genetics seem to play an influential—but not determinant—role in the condition. Approximately 4 percent of direct relatives of an IC patient (parents, siblings, or children) also have the condition; the odds are not much higher than the chances in the general population. In studies with identical twins with the same DNA, about half of the twins shared the diagnosis with their sibling while the other half did not.

There are many conditions that medical research still hasn't completely explained, and IC is one of them: It's likely that a comprehensive understanding of interstitial cystitis is decades away. In the meantime, stay informed of new research, but don't let the unknown slow your pace in finding what helps you right now.

Who Has IC?

The number of people with IC is shockingly high. The best population-based studies estimate more than twelve million people in the United States alone have the condition—which means it's about as common as coronary heart disease and depression, and more of a risk than Alzheimer's disease and type 1 diabetes. Overall, more than 5 percent of Americans are estimated to have interstitial cystitis.

The vast majority of those with interstitial cystitis may not be aware of the name for their symptoms. A survey of more than 130,000 households indicated that as many as 90 percent of people with the condition had not received a formal diagnosis, despite having seen more than three different doctors about

Just a few years later, a different group of researchers proposed scrapping the IC/PBS label in favor of Bladder Pain Syndrome. In Japan, scientists began using the name Hypersensitive Bladder Syndrome (HBS), shifting the emphasis away from pain and toward the urinary symptoms. Another definition proposes to place interstitial cystitis and chronic prostatitis (which some researchers believe to be the same condition) under the umbrella term Urologic Chronic Pelvic Pain Syndrome (UCPPS).

With all these proposed names being bandied about, the distinctions that researchers were trying to make have been lost, and the names have become essentially synonymous.

their symptoms. Less than half had any diagnosis at all, even an incorrect one. The prevalence of IC is much higher than most medical practitioners realize, and many patients go undiagnosed for years because of this misinformation.

How Is IC Diagnosed?

Interstitial cystitis is diagnosed by excluding all other explanations of the symptoms: that is, through a process of elimination. The American Urological Association uses the phrase "in the absence of infection or other identifiable cause." The initial suspect will be a urinary tract infection (UTI), which is caused by bacteria in the bladder or urinary tract. Even if the tests for a UTI come back negative, many doctors will still prescribe a course of antibiotics to patients. An IC diagnosis is only considered after an infection is ruled out, either by a negative diagnostic test or an ineffective round of antibiotics. Many physicians will also want to rule out bladder cancer as a possible cause of the pain, although the cause is seven to twenty times more likely to be IC than cancer.

Typically interstitial cystitis isn't diagnosed until the patient is in his or her forties. However, recent research suggests the onset of symptoms occurs much earlier, typically in the patient's twenties. A mistaken belief that IC doesn't manifest until middle age may make it even more difficult for younger patients to obtain a correct diagnosis.

IC and the Pelvic Floor Connection

The pelvic floor is the setting for IC. It houses the bladder and urethra, as well as the sexual organs and rectum. Pelvic floor muscles are responsible for urinating and defecating, sexual function, supporting the bladder, and stabilizing your body when you're moving or standing.

Interstitial cystitis is deeply interrelated with all these muscles, nerves, tissues, and functions of the pelvic floor. Tight muscles in the pelvic floor can be the underlying cause of many IC symptoms. Knots, or trigger points, in these muscles cause pain, bladder irritation, and urinary urgency. IC always affects your pelvic floor in some way; addressing the pelvic floor muscles is essential to successfully treating the condition.

Food Sensitivity and IC

One unique aspect of interstitial cystitis is the food sensitivity experienced by nearly 90 percent of patients. Certain foods and beverages—known as "triggers"—can substantially worsen symptoms. A relatively small number of food categories are the primary culprits. They include caffeine, alcohol, artificial sweeteners, spicy foods, and citrus fruits. Some patients find they are highly sensitive to what they eat and drink, while others only have to forego a few specific items. The different food triggers don't seem to have much in common with one another, and no conclusive explanation of the dietary connection has been proven, but making changes to your diet can result in major improvement in your condition.

Interstitial Cystitis in Men

Men manifest with the same symptoms, severity, and prevalence of interstitial cystitis. Interstitial cystitis has been known as a condition that primarily strikes women, but that assumption is based on research that's decades old. In fact, the latest research is finding that men are nearly as likely to have interstitial cystitis as women. Large, population-based studies show that 6.5 percent of women and 4.6 percent of men have interstitial cystitis symptoms. Plus, many researchers now believe that chronic prostatitis, diagnosed exclusively in men, may actually be the same condition as interstitial cystitis. If this is confirmed, it would make the prevalence almost identical between men and women.

Treatments are the same for men and women, and other chapters note whether there are any important differences between the genders in the studies. All of this means the vast majority of IC information is applicable to both men and women.

Associated Conditions

IC is associated with an increased risk of many other conditions. Researchers are trying to determine whether there is an underlying cause that unites many of these conditions, or if there is a cause-and-effect relationship. Patients with interstitial cystitis are at higher risk for irritable bowel syndrome (IBS), fibromyalgia, allergies and asthma, migraines, depression, and coronary heart disease. If you are diagnosed with interstitial cystitis, be vigilant about these other conditions and take appropriate actions to mitigate the effects they may have on your IC symptoms and your overall health.

Mental Health

Many members of the medical community are reluctant to mention the importance of mental health when dealing with interstitial cystitis—and for good reason, too. For decades, the symptoms of IC were trivialized and misdiagnosed as "women's hysteria" or another psychosomatic condition. That belief has been frustratingly slow to recede, and many patients, especially women, still bear the stigma of a perceived psychiatric, rather than physical, problem.

Addressing the mental health component of IC doesn't deny the physical condition: It acknowledges that chronic pain has an effect on the mind and on emotional health. Studies have shown that chronic pain can rewire the brain. Over time, it actually begins to expect painful sensations. Patients with chronic conditions, including IC, are at higher risk for depression, suicidal thoughts, and anxiety. The good news is that taking steps to address mental and emotional health can help reduce pain and other physical symptoms while restoring a sense of control to your life.

Takeaways

- **No one will care as much about your health as you do.** Take control of your own health. IC is a complex condition, and will require a holistic approach to treatment. Many myths and much misinformation can hinder a proper diagnosis and treatment. Educate yourself about the condition and pay attention to your own body. Healing is a journey, and relief is possible.

- **Your journey is made up of many small steps.** Take a step forward each day. If you do, you'll be shocked when you look back at how far you've come. Onward!

2

IC and You:

Symptoms of IC

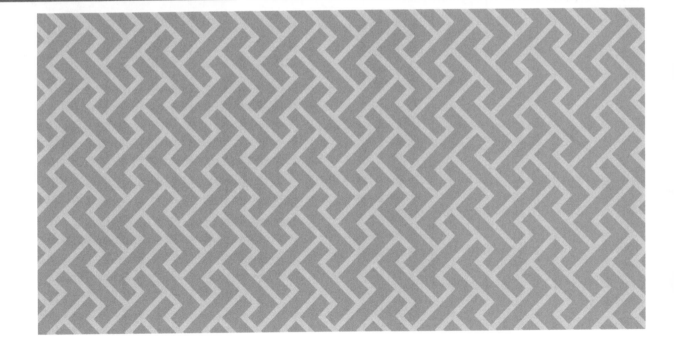

Interstitial cystitis is a complex condition, and can manifest in many ways. Patients can present with just a few, most, or all of the symptoms outlined in this chapter. The condition is characterized by pain, pressure, or discomfort that seems to be related to the bladder. Nearly all IC patients experience frequent and urgent urination. Most also report some kind of pelvic pain (suprapubic, abdominal, or groin) associated with the condition.

Of course, this doesn't mean that recognizing IC symptoms is simple. Put yourself in your doctor's lab coat for a moment. (Now that you've read this far, you probably have about as much knowledge of the condition as most medical students do upon graduation.) You've seen three patients this morning, and your task is to decide which patient has interstitial cystitis.

- Your first patient is a forty-seven-year-old man. He has noticed he uses the bathroom more often as he gets older, and that it takes a longer time to start a stream of urine. His biggest complaint is testicular and groin pain after sex.

- Your second patient is a twenty-four-year-old woman who has just graduated from college. She's physically fit—a former soccer player—and seems to be the epitome of health. But she gets up at night to go to the bathroom and has noticed she goes to the bathroom about fifteen times a day. She has been diagnosed with several urinary tract infections (UTI) over the past few months, which didn't improve with antibiotics, and she has a sharp, stabbing pain in her lower abdomen.

- Your third patient is a sixty-three-year-old woman whose primary complaint is severe low back pain, which started after she had her first child more than twenty years ago. She's noticed the pain gets worse when her bladder is full or when she is constipated, and eating spicy foods tends to cause a burning sensation when she urinates.

Which patient has interstitial cystitis? The answer is *all of them*. And these are just some of the ways in which IC manifests.

PATIENT SYMPTOM SUMMARY

	Patient 1	Patient 2	Patient 3
Age	47	24	63
Gender	Male	Female	Female
Chief complaint	Testicular pain after sex	Frequent and urgent urination	Low back pain
Other information	It often takes a long time to urinate, and frequency of bathroom use has increased as he gets older.	Reports of lower abdominal pain and frequent urinary tract infections	Sometimes gets a burning sensation with urination after eating spicy foods

IC or a UTI?

The symptoms of interstitial cystitis are almost identical to those of urinary tract infections, and nearly all IC patients begin their medical journey incorrectly diagnosed with a UTI. A bacterial infection of the urinary tract or bladder can cause the symptoms of urgency and frequency of urination, burning in the urethra, and bladder pressure or pain. (For more information on the diagnosis of IC, and how to tell the difference between UTIs and IC, see chapter 4.)

Referred Pain

Some symptoms caused by IC can seem completely unrelated to the bladder or pelvic floor. This is known as *referred pain*, where the pain is experienced in a different part of the body, not the part that actually hurts. Many patients report lower back or hip pain, and may not even realize it's caused by their interstitial cystitis. Referred pain like this is the result of irritated nerves in the pelvic floor. When they are disturbed—which happens often in IC—the pain can manifest anywhere the nerve reaches.

There are two main reasons for referred pain. When the muscles of the pelvic floor become tight, they can squeeze and irritate the nerves that run through the pelvis. These tight spots, or trigger points, can cause pain anywhere along the length of the nerve—in the same way that a tight muscle in your neck can cause a headache.

referred pain: Pain or discomfort experienced at a location in the body other than its true source.

The bladder itself may also be irritated. Nerves connect to organs, such as the bladder, and link to other areas of the body. When organs experience problems, pain can shoot down these connecting nerves to other body parts. This might seem odd at first, but you're probably already familiar with this phenomenon: For instance, it's why the first major symptoms of a heart attack are often pain in the left arm, jaw, or back. There's nothing physically wrong with the arm or jaw, but they manifest the pain radiating from the damaged heart. The same kind of pain is experienced during menstruation. No one is actually punching you in the back, but it feels that way as a result of the pain referred from the uterus.

Just like the heart, uterus, and other organs, the bladder also has a pain referral pattern. It commonly causes pain directly above its location in the lower abdomen (suprapubic pain), a few inches (centimeters) below the belly button, but the pain can also radiate to the inner thighs or even the tailbone. As you'd expect, improving the condition of the bladder can alleviate the pain in the inner thighs—but, in an interesting twist, improving the condition of the inner thighs can actually reduce pain and symptoms in the bladder.

Thanks to these interconnections in the body, addressing one apparently unrelated area can have a major benefit on other symptoms. This is a big deal! Who would have guessed that working to alleviate tightness and inflammation in the legs or stomach could reduce your urinary urgency and frequency? This is why your bladder symptoms may improve from such things as stretching, deep breathing, a warm bath, and other treatments that don't target the bladder itself.

Nervous System Upregulation

The bladder has the highest nerve density of any organ. Most of these nerves are considered "silent" and don't typically pass on information or pain sensations to the brain. However, if they are constantly stimulated, like they are in IC patients, these nerves become active and start to transmit signals. With all these formerly silent nerves firing at once, it's no wonder that IC patients often experience extremely high levels of pain and constant urges to urinate. Once these nerves become overly sensitized, it is difficult to return them to their natural, silent state; this is one of the main reasons it can take a long time to treat IC symptoms effectively.

This issue of nerve upregulation and hypersensitivity is important to understand. If we heard from all of our nerves all the time, we would go mad. Imagine sorting out sensations from every part of the body at the same time! Thankfully, most nerves have a threshold. They fire off a report to the brain only when the pressure exceeds a certain level. That's why you aren't conscious of your jeans brushing against your shins all day long, but slamming your knee into the sharp corner of the coffee table results in howls of pain.

 The Nature of Pain

Pain is a good thing.

That may sound counterintuitive, but the fact is that pain serves a vital function in our lives. It's the body's way of reporting a problem and forcing us to take corrective action. Here's how it works: Your body is laced with nerve receptors that have a simple job. When they register a sensation, they activate, sending a message that's passed through the body to the spinal cord and, ultimately, to the brain.

The brain is then responsible for interpreting that signal. If it believes the report is trivial, the brain can turn down its sensitivity and ignore those reports. But, if it believes the information is important, it can amplify the "volume" of the signal.

Part of the challenge of chronic pain conditions, such as interstitial cystitis, is the brain is primed to receive these reports of pain, a phenomenon called nervous system upregulation. Reversing this upregulation by taking medication for pain relief, eliminating pelvic floor triggers causing the constant pain signals, or reducing stress and anxiety, can help calm the entire nervous system. This can be a major challenge for IC patients, but it can be incredibly beneficial in reducing pain levels.

Chronic pain lasting more than three months can reduce the threshold at which pain is reported to the brain. When this threshold level is lowered, stimuli we wouldn't normally notice are reported to the brain. We've all experienced examples of this. Typically, you don't notice a light brush against your skin, but if you've just walked through a spider web, you notice everything: You're convinced every breeze, every clothing tag, and every stray hair is actually the spider crawling over your skin. The same thing happens when you watch a horror movie. Normally, the sensation of a hand on your shoulder doesn't make you jump out of your skin and scream, but it does when you hear ominous music and watch the heroine descend into the unlit basement.

This is what often happens with chronic pain and interstitial cystitis. The nerves become so used to firing, and the brain becomes so used to receiving those pain signals, that the threshold for pain is lowered. Gentle sensations you wouldn't normally notice are now reported to your brain as pain. This is "upregulation" of the nervous system.

This upregulation has many consequences. You can experience hypersensitivity as the bladder fills: Your nerves report that the bladder is already full and needs to be emptied, even if you know you just did a few minutes ago. The referring nerves that connect from the bladder to the pelvic region can also be hypersensitive, causing suprapubic tenderness that can make even light contact with the waistband of pants or skirts excruciating. Finally, pelvic floor dysfunction as the result of IC can cause the pelvic nerves to be overstimulated as well, referring pain throughout the pelvic floor and causing additional symptoms, such as lower back pain, tailbone pain, pain with sex, and urinary symptoms. (For more information on the intricate connection between the bladder and pelvic floor, see chapter 5.)

Reversing the nervous system upregulation is among the most important aspects of treating interstitial cystitis. Restoring the nerves to their normal function and stopping the hypersensitivity can reduce symptoms greatly. It's likely the nerves have been irritated for a long time—probably before you began to experience symptoms—so it can also take some time for them to calm down. Once they do, stimuli that used to be painful or irritating may not even be noticed.

Common Symptoms of Interstitial Cystitis

As we saw with the three sample patients earlier in this chapter, IC is challenging to diagnose and manage because everyone experiences it differently. Some symptoms are common among almost all patients, but others vary widely. In one study of nearly 300 patients, researchers examined the most prevalent symptoms. The four most common and severe were:

1. Suprapubic pain
2. Frequency of urination
3. Urgency of urination
4. Nocturnia (waking at night to urinate)

SYMPTOMS AND SEVERITY

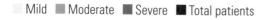 Mild ■ Moderate ■ Severe ■ Total patients

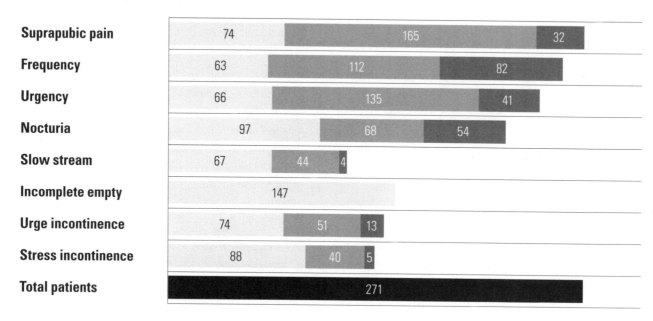

Suprapubic pain — 74 | 165 | 32

Frequency — 63 | 112 | 82

Urgency — 66 | 135 | 41

Nocturia — 97 | 68 | 54

Slow stream — 67 | 44 | 4

Incomplete empty — 147

Urge incontinence — 74 | 51 | 13

Stress incontinence — 88 | 40 | 5

Total patients — 271

Results from a survey of 271 IC patients who were asked what symptoms they experienced and whether they were mild, moderate, or severe. The numbers stated represent the portion of the total number of patients examined (271) who exhibited a particular symptom. For example, 74 of the 271 patients surveyed had mild suprapubic pain, 165 had moderate pain, and 32 described it as severe; all patients had some suprapubic pain. Source: Al-Zahrani, A., and J. Gajewski. "Long-Term Efficacy and Tolerability of Pentosan Polysuphate Sodium in the Treatment of Bladder Pain Syndrome," *Canadian Urological Association Journal* 5, no. 2 (April 2011): 113–18.

Urinary Symptoms

Interstitial cystitis is a combination of urinary symptoms and pain symptoms.

■ Frequency of Urination

A typical adult will urinate four to six times daily, so frequency can be considered a symptom if urination occurs more than seven times per day. Almost 95 percent of patients report increased frequency of urination. Patients with this symptom may be tempted to rationalize it away with excuses such as, "I drink a lot of water," "I'm going just in case," or "I must have a small bladder." But consistently using the bathroom seven or more times daily is considered a symptom.

■ Urgency of Urination

Urgency is the sudden and powerful need to urinate. This symptom of IC is almost as common as increased frequency, and these symptoms are often seen and referred to together. If the urge is powerful enough it can cause urge incontinence, in which urine actually escapes. Keep in mind it should take at least ten seconds to void a full bladder. If your bladder empties in less time, it wasn't full, and you are experiencing urinary urgency.

■ Nocturia

Nocturia is urgent and frequent urination that occurs at night. Urinating two or more times each night is considered abnormal, and is a symptom shared by nearly 80 percent of IC patients. Hypersensitivity to bladder filling can be a culprit here. The bladder continually fills throughout the night. Typically we don't notice this until it is full, when we get the signal to wake up and go. However, if your bladder is extremely sensitive to any sort of sensation, the slow trickle of urine into the bladder can be enough that the body interprets it as the "wake up and go" signal.

■ Hesitancy and Decreased Urine Flow

The unfortunate contradiction for many IC patients is they experience an irresistible urge to use the bathroom, but once they arrive it can be very difficult to go. The flow can either be slow to start or weak once it has begun. This can occur for a variety of reasons.

If the bladder sends the signal that it needs to go even though it is nearly empty, there just isn't much to void. Hesitancy can also be due to tight muscles in the pelvic floor. If they're unable to relax fully, it's more difficult for urine to pass through. Finally, in a vicious cycle, the anxiety regarding bathroom use that many IC patients experience can also contribute to this symptom. More than 40 percent of patients reported urinary hesitancy. In men, this is often blamed on the prostate, but it is a common problem with interstitial cystitis.

■ Incomplete Voiding of the Bladder

Closely related to urgency and frequency is the feeling that the bladder is never quite empty, regardless of how many times you urinate. It can be hard to determine whether this feeling arises because there's actually urine left in the bladder, or because you experience the urge to go again immediately after you've finished.

Leftover urine can be due to tight muscles in the pelvic floor that make it difficult to void the bladder completely. Your bladder may not be doing a good job of contracting to get the remaining urine out when it's nearly empty. Or it could just be your perception: Your bladder may actually be empty, but the hypersensitive nerves report a different story. More than half of IC patients report the feeling of incomplete voiding as a symptom.

■ *Bladder Pressure*

A feeling of tightness or compression of the bladder, this pressure is also described as a continual sensation of a full bladder. It can be accompanied by pain or pressure in the pubic region a few inches (centimeters) below the belly button. Some patients who experience this pressure may not be properly diagnosed with IC because they don't report it as pain. However, the truth is that pressure or discomfort qualify for an IC diagnosis and may eventually become even more painful if left untreated.

■ *Incontinence*

While incontinence isn't a classic symptom, it can be present in IC patients due to pelvic floor dysfunction. Stress incontinence occurs when an outside force—such as laughing, sneezing, coughing, or lifting something heavy—places pressure on the bladder area and triggers incontinence.

Urge incontinence is the uncontrollable need to release urine. It can be the end result of the urgency felt by many patients. The bladder may spasm and push out urine the pelvic floor is unable to hold back. Pelvic floor dysfunction and weak pelvic floor muscles contribute to this symptom. Half of IC patients reported at least occasional incontinence when asked about their symptoms.

Pain Symptoms

Pain or discomfort is required for an IC diagnosis. Urinary symptoms without pain may be caused by an overactive bladder or another condition, but pain is the hallmark symptom of IC.

■ *Suprapubic Pain*

All IC patients surveyed reported at least mild suprapubic pain, centered a few inches (centimeters) below the belly button and directly above the bladder. In some cases, the region can be so tender that even waistband pressure can be unbearable. This is a standard location for referred bladder pain, and often increases with a filling bladder. Part of the increased frequency of the condition may be due to the body's attempts to keep the bladder empty to prevent this discomfort.

■ *Bladder or Urethral Pain*

This pain can be a very intense, localized around the bladder or in the urethra. Patients have described it as a twisting knife, an acidic kind of burning, or the feeling that there is ground glass in the bladder and urethra.

■ *Pain or Burning Related to Urination*

Urethral burning, either during or after urination, is a common symptom of interstitial cystitis. Some researchers believe it is caused by damage to the lining of the urethra or the bladder, which allows toxins in the urine to penetrate and burn. It can also be caused by dysfunction in the pelvic floor muscles, which irritates the nerves and muscles that control the urethra.

■ *Pelvic Pain*

Pelvic pain can manifest in many ways and in many locations in IC patients. For women, it can present in the vagina, perineum, or rectum, either on the surface or deeper inside. Men can experience pain in the penis, scrotum/testicles, perineum, or rectum. Tight or overactive pelvic floor muscles resulting from IC are often the culprits behind pelvic pain.

■ *Lower Back, Hip, Groin, or Tailbone Pain*

Pain can also be referred to other sites in the pelvic region. Patients often report discomfort in the lower back or hip, but pain around the tailbone, groin, or upper legs is also common. This is usually referred pain from the nerves and muscle trigger points from the pelvic floor that have become overly sensitized as a result of the condition. Groin and inner thigh pain can be referred directly from the bladder itself.

■ *Pain with Sex (Dyspareunia)*

Studies have shown that a majority of women with IC experience pain during or after sexual intercourse. This can present as pain directly in the vagina, urethra, or bladder— or sometimes all three. This pain can linger for several days after intercourse.

Men report testicular, urethral, or penile pain, as well as bladder pain, with erection or ejaculation. A burning sensation at the tip of the penis is also common. Pain surrounding intercourse for men is not as well known or researched as it is in women, but can be just as impactful and disruptive. Pain with sex is a classic symptom of pelvic floor dysfunction.

Symptom Log

Recording your symptoms in a daily log can be extremely useful, especially in the early months of the condition. This log is for your reference and for sharing with your physician. Doctors can be dismissive of statements such as, "It feels like there's ground glass in my bladder," especially if there is no evidence of bacterial infection to offer an easy explanation. It's much harder to ignore a written symptom log that chronicles various symptoms and pain levels over several weeks.

Plus, this log can be informative for you as a patient. You'll notice which activities, foods, or other factors influence your symptoms. Outside conditions that increase the symptoms are called triggers. Common triggers include:

- Changes in diet
- Changes in hormone levels during the monthly menstrual cycle
- Intensive exercise
- Prolonged sitting
- Sexual intercourse
- Stress

As you try different treatments, your symptom log will provide you with an objective way to determine whether you're improving.

Symptoms are clues to what's going on inside your body. Medical professionals use symptoms and patient experiences as essential parts of any diagnosis. Symptoms can vary over the course of a day or week; that's why it's crucial to track and understand them. They can help your healthcare team and guide your treatment. Whether you're just starting out and working toward a diagnosis or have had the condition for decades, a clear and concise symptom log can help make sense of a frustrating situation.

The following symptom log chronicles your symptoms over the course of a week. You'll give each major symptom a rating for the day (0 being no symptom at all; 10 being the worst you can imagine). Also, note the time of day when the symptom was the worst. If you notice any factors that had an effect, either positive or negative, on the symptom, write them down as well. For nocturia, write down the number of times you got up to use the bathroom during the previous night.

You'll also give your overall symptoms a rating for the day. This summary information helps you look back to see how far you've come over the course of treatment. Use the Notes section to document anything else you notice about your condition— actions that make your symptoms better or worse, changes to your activity level or diet, or anything else that might provide a clue.

SYMPTOM LOG

	MON	TUES	WED	THUR	FRI	SAT	SUN
Urgency/frequency							
(0 to 10)							
Worst time							
Affecting factors							
Suprapubic pain							
(0 to 10)							
Worst time							
Affecting factors							
Bladder pain							
(0 to 10)							
Worst time							
Affecting factors							
Other: _____							
(0 to 10)							
Worst time							
Affecting factors							
Nocturia (# of times)							
Overall day score (1 to 10)							
Notes (Examples include challenges, triumphs, things that help, or other pertinent information.)							

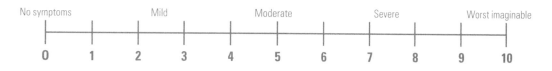

No symptoms Mild Moderate Severe Worst imaginable

0   1   2   3   4   5   6   7   8   9   10

A body map is a great resource that can help you, your doctor, or your physical therapist to visualize the symptoms of your condition. To use the map, just mark on the image the location of the pain. Note whether it is localized or spread out and do your best to accurately draw the pain sites on the front and back. This tool can be used to identify the type of pain as well; some patients will use different colors or labels to distinguish between a dull ache, burning, or a sharp pain.

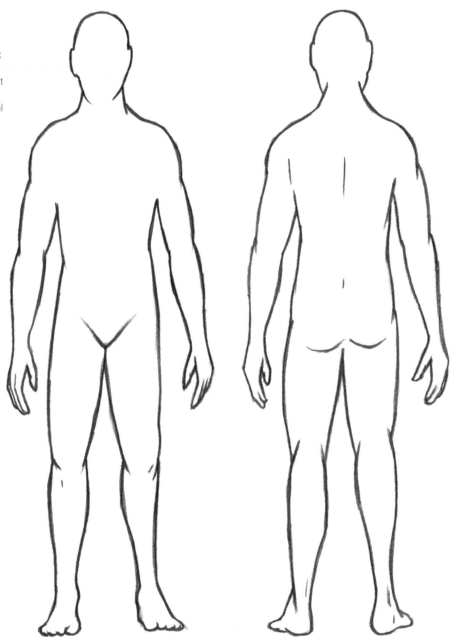

Another tool you can use to track your progress is the O'Leary-Sant symptom and problem indexes. This validated measurement tool assesses the overall symptoms of IC and how much they affect your daily life. This is a good tool to use monthly to track progress in your IC journey. Avoid looking at your answers to previous indexes before filling out a new one.

O'LEARY-SANT SYMPTOM AND PROBLEM INDEXES

IC symptom index	IC problem index
During the past month, how often have you felt the strong need to urinate with little or no warning? 0. ____ Not at all 1. ____ Less than 1 time in 5 2. ____ Less than half the time 3. ____ About half the time 4. ____ More than half the time 5. ____ Almost always	During the past month, how much has frequent urination during the day been a problem for you? 0. ____ Not a problem 1. ____ Very small problem 2. ____ Small problem 3. ____ Medium problem 4. ____ Big problem
During the past month, have you had to urinate less than two hours after you finished urinating? 0. ____ Not at all 1. ____ Less than 1 time in 5 2. ____ Less than half the time 3. ____ About half the time 4. ____ More than half the time 5. ____ Almost always	During the past month, how much has getting up at night to urinate been a problem for you? 0. ____ Not a problem 1. ____ Very small problem 2. ____ Small problem 3. ____ Medium problem 4. ____ Big problem

Source: O'Leary, M. P., G. R. Sant, F. J. Fowler, et al. "The Interstitial Cystitis Symptom Index and Problem Index," *Urology* 49. Supplement 5A: 58–63.

O'LEARY-SANT SYMPTOM AND PROBLEM INDEX *(continued)*

IC symptom index	IC problem index
During the past month, how often did you most typically get up at night to urinate?	During the past month, how much has needing to urinate with little warning been a problem for you?
0. _____ Not at all	0. _____ Not a problem
1. _____ Once per night	1. _____ Very small problem
2. _____ Two times per night	2. _____ Small problem
3. _____ Three times per night	3. _____ Medium problem
4. _____ Four times per night	4. _____ Big problem
5. _____ Five or more times per night	
During the past month, have you experienced pain or burning in your bladder?	During the past month, how much has burning, pain, discomfort, or pressure in your bladder been a problem for you?
0. _____ Not at all	0. _____ Not a problem
1. _____ A few times	1. _____ Very small problem
2. _____ Fairly often	2. _____ Small problem
3. _____ Usually	3. _____ Medium problem
4. _____ Almost always	4. _____ Big problem
Total: _____ *Add the numerical value of the checked entries*	**Total:** _____ *Add the numerical value of the checked entries*

O'Leary, Michael P., et al. "The Interstitial Cystitis Symptom Index and Problem Index." *Urology* 49, no. 5, Supplement 1 (May 1997): 58–63.

IC and Associated Conditions

One of the challenges IC patients face is the condition puts them at an increased risk for other medical problems. It's unclear whether there is a common underlying reason for these issues, but any other medical conditions need to be properly managed or they can derail your IC progress.

Don't be overwhelmed by the information on associated conditions—much of it may not be relevant to you at all. And it's likely there are dozens of other risk factors for each condition that are significantly more important than the IC connection. Not everyone with IC will have an associated condition, and the risk for many of these is relatively low. Simply be aware of the increased risk and work proactively to manage it. When you're on the IC journey, these associated conditions can be like a pebble that sneaks into your hiking boot. You may be eager to push forward, but every step is dogged by the presence of that annoying little stone. It's worth taking the time to pull off your boot and remove it.

CONDITIONS PRESENT WITH IC

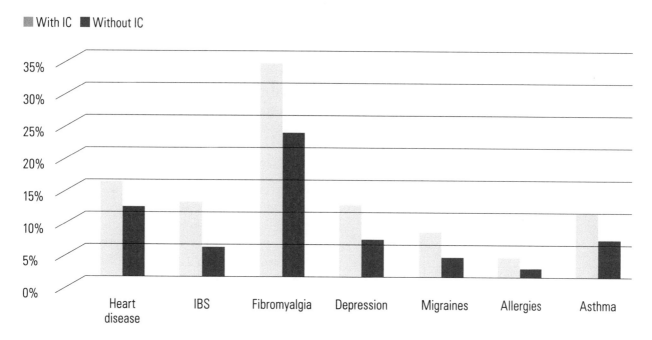

In a 2013 study, the authors reviewed data from more than 700 women diagnosed with interstitial cystitis. They compared the prevalence of other conditions against members of the general population to determine which are most strongly associated with an interstitial cystitis diagnosis. Source: Chung, S-D, S-P Liu, C-C Li, H-C Lin. "Bladder Pain Syndrome/Interstitial Cystitis Is Associated with Hyperthyroidism," *PLOS ONE* 8(8): e72284, 2013.

IC and Irritable Bowel Syndrome

The link between IC and Irritable Bowel Syndrome (IBS) is one of the strongest connections reported, and the average age of onset for both IC and IBS is nearly identical. IBS presents as either constipation-dominant or diarrhea-dominant.

An obvious common denominator between these conditions is the effect of diet on symptoms. Dietary changes are a crucial part of dealing with IC—90 percent of patients have symptoms related to food sensitivity—and they can be equally important to the proper management of IBS.

IC and IBS are also both highly affected by the pelvic floor muscles and dysfunction. The small intestine is coiled in the gut below the rib cage and is the true source of "stomach-aches." It's also in close proximity to the bladder and pelvic floor. Irritation in the bowels causes inflammation, which can tighten the abdominal muscles and fascia in the pelvic area. Not only can this disrupt normal bowel function further, but it can also make your bladder even angrier. In this way, the irritability of your IBS can contribute to your bladder irritation.

Many patients see dramatic improvements in their IBS symptoms when the pelvic floor causes of their IC symptoms are treated, and vice versa. There is clearly a pelvic floor connection between the two conditions, and it can be addressed and managed to help both conditions.

 irritable bowel syndrome (IBS): A group of symptoms that include pain or discomfort in the abdomen and changes in bowel movement patterns.

IC, Fibromyalgia, and Chronic Fatigue Syndrome

Fibromyalgia causes widespread tenderness and muscle pain, often located at specific points within the body. Fatigue, waking up unrefreshed in the morning, and cognitive or memory problems are also considered for a diagnosis. These symptoms must be present for at least three months at a similar level of severity to be considered fibromyalgia.

Chronic fatigue syndrome (CFS) is defined by generalized fatigue lasting longer than six months that doesn't improve with additional rest. With a major symptom of fatigue in common, fibromyalgia and chronic fatigue syndrome are heavily interrelated: Researchers believe more than 70 percent of fibromyalgia patients meet the criteria for CFS.

Like IC, there is no routine lab or diagnostic test that can conclusively yield a fibromyalgia or chronic fatigue syndrome diagnosis. There's definitely a connection between IC and these conditions—more than 35 percent of patients with IC may have one or both of them. Plus, both IC and fibromyalgia/CFS are chronic pain syndromes, and some researchers have suggested that IC can actually progress into the multiple pain sites of fibromyalgia if left untreated.

Still, don't assume you have fibromyalgia or CFS because you seem to fit the symptom list. A rheumatologist can help you properly diagnose and start treatment if appropriate; proper treatment of fibromyalgia or CFS-related pain or fatigue can significantly help your IC symptoms by working to break the pain cycle.

 fibromyalgia: Chronic disorder characterized by widespread musculoskeletal pain, fatigue, and tenderness in localized areas.

If you have both IC and fibromyalgia or CFS, address each condition to the best of your ability. Anything you can do to shut down the bombardment of pain receptors in your body from fibromyalgia will help your body to break the cycle of pain associated with IC—and vice versa.

IC, Asthma, and Allergies

Patients with IC have been shown to have an increased risk for both asthma and allergies. Though the causal link, if any, is unknown, there can be implications for your IC treatment if you also struggle with either of these other conditions.

Some consequences of allergies—coughing, sneezing, and blowing your nose—involve violent movements of your pelvic floor and can further irritate these tight muscles.

Asthma or allergies can also result in a habit of shallow breathing. Quick, shallow breaths are associated with stressful situations, so constantly breathing in this way can amplify the effects of anxiety and stress. Deep breathing, using your diaphragm, actually relaxes the pelvic floor.

Another danger is that asthma and allergies can limit activities and exercise or disrupt your sleep at a time when rest is critical. Work to get your allergies and asthma under control, and don't let the conditions hinder your recovery.

 allergy: Damaging immune response by the body to a substance, especially pollen, fur, a particular food, or dust, to which it has become hypersensitive.

Takeaways

- **Symptoms of IC vary widely from patient to patient.** Almost all IC patients have some sort of pain or discomfort that's perceived to be bladder related, along with urinary symptoms, such as urgency and frequency. However, patients also experience many other symptoms, such as pain in the suprapubic area, lower back, hip, and groin. The majority of IC patients have pain with sex; other urinary symptoms, such as burning with urination or urinary retention, are also common. There is no "normal" set of IC symptoms—they are unique to each patient.

- **Symptoms are signposts on your IC journey.** The symptoms of interstitial cystitis can range from irritating to debilitating. I encourage my patients to view these symptoms as signposts, or clues. By paying attention to your body and keeping a symptom log, you can begin to understand what affects your condition. Soon you'll be able to look back at your symptom log and—just like a signpost on a trail—see exactly how far you've come or where you need to go on your healing journey.

3

THE CAUSE CONUNDRUM:

What We Know

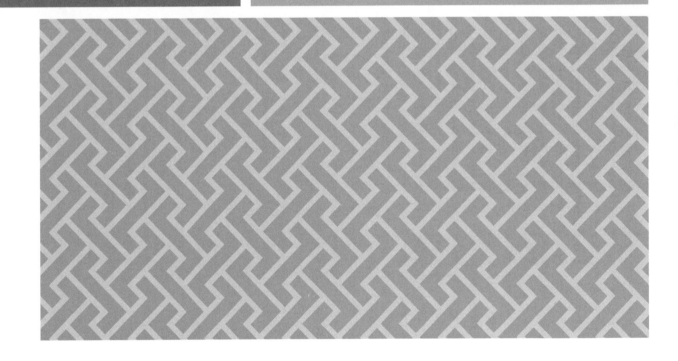

Although many theories have been proposed, researchers still haven't been able to pinpoint the cause(s) of interstitial cystitis. And, as of right now, none of the possible explanations is particularly helpful for you as the patient *or* for your practitioners. Some researchers postulate that IC is caused by damage to the bladder lining, allowing urine to come into contact with the sensitive tissue underneath. Others have explored dysfunction or disease in the nerves that innervate the bladder and urethra. The immune system may also play an important role, almost like it would in an allergy or autoimmune disorder. And the pelvic floor is intimately connected with all facets of the condition.

The root cause of IC may be one of these factors, or a combination of them. Or it may be something completely different—something scientists have yet to identify. Studying the underlying cause of IC is a logical place to start to find an answer or a cure: Determining its origin may be the first step toward finding a universal treatment or preventing the condition entirely. Unfortunately, its cause remains elusive and it may be decades before a consensus emerges and is fully proven. The fact that we haven't yet found a single theory that could potentially explain the entire condition, or a single treatment that works in the majority of patients, certainly indicates the answer is not likely to be a simple one. So, this chapter provides a synopsis of what we do and do not know about IC.

The important thing to realize for both patients and practitioners is interstitial cystitis causes a feedback loop that begins to amplify the symptoms of the condition. An initial injury occurs—regardless of the root cause—and causes pain and bladder irritation. The bladder deals with discomfort by trying to flush the system, creating the urge to urinate. As the problems persist, many of those "silent" nerves in the pelvis begin to communicate, reporting pain and discomfort. The tissue in the area becomes inflamed and tender, which causes more pain, which activates more silent nerves, until the entire system is engulfed in the recurring loop.

It is essential to realize this cycle must be broken for healing to take place—and that is why there is no quick cure for IC. This cycle may have been building for months or even years before symptoms finally surfaced, and it can take an equally long time to restore those nerves to their silent state—and to regain normal function, reduce inflammation, and alleviate pain.

Additionally, we know IC is accompanied by pelvic floor muscle spasm, which is a tightness of the pelvis muscles that support the bladder and surround the urethra. (For more on IC and the pelvic floor, see chapter 5.) It is unclear whether this muscle spasm is a result of or a cause of interstitial cystitis. In either case, it must be treated to break the cycle of the condition. Dysfunction in the pelvic floor can be a primary cause of IC symptoms for many patients.

Regardless of the origin of IC, you can successfully treat and manage the condition. Just because researchers haven't been able to isolate a single root cause doesn't mean we don't know a great deal about IC. Because the cause is so ambiguous, it can be tempting to "lock into" one explanation or another (especially if you're a hyperfocused type of person), but don't limit your treatment options based on what you believe the cause of your IC to be.

"Interstitial cystitis cannot be addressed entirely by focusing on the bladder lining alone."

A Problem with the Bladder's Lining?

The theory of damage to the bladder lining has been a primary focus of IC research for more than one hundred years. As you've read, early work in the field focused on lesions that form in the bladder of some patients, as well as small wounds in the bladder known as glomerulations.

This theory is tantalizingly simple: Cracks or wounds in the bladder lining allow urine to penetrate into the sensitive skin underneath and cause irritation. The bladder responds by trying to flush away the irritant, explaining the urgency and frequency of urination in interstitial cystitis. The discomfort and inflammation in the bladder refer pain to the suprapubic region above the bladder. The irritated bladder negatively affects the pelvic floor, which can be responsible for additional symptoms.

By now you should know to be wary of answers this simple when it comes to IC, and there's lots of contradictory evidence around this theory. Supporters point to the effect diet can have on IC symptoms: Removing bladder irritants, such as caffeine, spicy foods, and citrus, has been shown to have a positive effect in nearly 90 percent of IC patients. The potassium sensitivity test was deliberately designed to introduce an irritant to the bladder to see how patients respond. A potassium-rich solution is instilled directly into the bladder; for most people, it causes no irritation at all, but, in IC patients, it causes excruciating pain. So that confirms it, right?

Not so fast. Only about 80 percent of IC patients experience pain with the potassium sensitivity test. If IC really is due to a leaky bladder lining, how is it possible that many patients with IC do not experience pain when an irritant is delivered directly to the bladder? Foods high in potassium, such as bananas, have been shown to be some of the safest foods for IC patients to eat. And researchers have shown that urine's acidity—which we'd expect to be a major source of irritation if the condition were solely due to a leaky bladder lining—doesn't affect symptoms in IC patients.

Treatments that protect the bladder and reinforce the bladder lining do work in some patients, but are ineffective in many others. Perhaps the most compelling piece of contradictory evidence to this theory is what happens when the bladder is removed completely—many patients continue to have symptoms of interstitial cystitis.

There have been dozens of studies on IC bladders, in both human patients and animal models. Many try to identify any differences between "normal" and IC bladders. Some researchers have found differences in the types of proteins embedded in the bladder's lining of animal models that may make it more permeable to urine. Other studies found differences in the interstitial bladder cells themselves that would make them more susceptible to irritation. Still others reported differences in the amounts of acid-sensing ion channels in the bladders of IC patients. The trouble is researchers do not consistently find a single potential cause, and are often unable to reproduce their findings.

Although research may eventually identify additional risk factors for IC related to the bladder lining, or may find a singular cause related to a porous bladder, IC cannot be addressed entirely by focusing on the bladder lining alone.

Is IC Hereditary?

Some research has demonstrated that the condition has a genetic component, but the most recent studies have shown only 4 percent of first-degree family members (parents, siblings, or children) were also diagnosed with IC, which is not substantially higher than in the rest of the population.

One of the best ways to evaluate the genetic component of a condition is to look at sets of identical twins: They share the same DNA, so a genetic connection should be very clear. For example, in a condition such as Huntington's disease, which is completely determined by genes, if one twin has the condition, the other is certain to have it. But, when researchers evaluated pairs of identical twins for IC, approximately half shared an IC diagnosis, while the other half did not.

Other studies investigating more specialized aspects of the condition, such as Hunner's ulcers (lesions) or slight differences in the bladder lining, have shown potential gender-based genetic links, but none of this research has yet proved conclusive. Overall, it does look as if there is a genetic component to interstitial cystitis, but it is not nearly as pronounced as in many other conditions. Ultimately, genetics is not destiny: Although a family history of the condition may increase your chances of having it, it's certainly not a guarantee.

Does Inflammation Cause IC?

Inflammation has an important function in the body. When working properly, the inflammatory response acts like a paramedic rushing to a roadside accident. As a first responder, it races to the scene of an injury to address the cause of the problem, remove damaged cells, and jumpstart healing. Swelling, redness, and skin that is warm to the touch are signs of inflammation and can be present with everything from infections to a sprained ankle. Once the acute cause of the problem is removed, the inflammation usually fades away.

However, conditions can arise when the inflammatory system is overactive. Asthma, allergies, rheumatoid arthritis, and many other autoimmune diseases involve a heightened inflammatory response, and there's evidence this system may be out of whack in many patients with IC. Research has revealed an increase in inflammatory molecules (mast cells, cytokines, or C-reactive protein markers) in patients. And when present for a long time, as with chronic illness, inflammation can heighten pain and impede function. Specifically, inflammation in the bladder has been correlated with increased urinary urgency and pain.

One question facing researchers, then, is the classic chicken-or-egg conundrum: Is the inflammation causing the pain or is the inflammation a natural response to pain that's already there? Either way, there is clearly a feedback loop at work. The symptoms prompt inflammation that lingers and causes additional pain, which again calls for more inflammation in the region to try to resolve the problem. A successful treatment program must focus on relieving this cycle of pain and inflammation.

How Does IC Affect the Brain?

What does the brain have to do with a bladder and pelvic condition, such as interstitial cystitis? Well, the brain is responsible for translating the electrical signals from your bladder nerves into the knowledge that the bladder is full and needs to be emptied. But with IC, the brain interprets sensations of pain or urinary urgency instead. One of the first hypotheses about IC was that it was due to a nervous tic in the bladder—the result of nerves firing uncontrollably.

Recent advances in brain-imaging technology have offered new insight into the matter. In a 2014 study funded by the National Institutes of Health, researchers discovered differences in the brains of people with IC, particularly in the regions that process pain, the sensation of touch, and pain's emotional components. Because the brain is flexible and can change in response to repeated stimuli, it's hard to know whether these differences contribute to IC or if the brain has been rewired by the chronic pain that accompanies IC. That important issue remains to be tested, and no verdict has been reached. This connection with the brain is important, and it helps explain why some treatments that address emotional stressors or work to retrain the brain can reduce the pain and symptoms associated with IC.

Upregulation of the Nervous System: How High Is Your Volume Set?

Some of the most recent research focuses on the nervous system responses of people with IC. The nervous system is divided into two major categories: the somatic (the voluntary system) and the autonomic (the automatic system).

The autonomic system has two systems that are essentially "volume knobs" for the nerves: the sympathetic and the parasympathetic nervous systems. The sympathetic "fight or flight" system cranks the volume up, while the parasympathetic "rest and relax" system turns the volume down. In a normal person, these two systems should work together in harmony, ensuring the music of the nerves is playing at an audible, but not deafening, level.

Some studies have shown, though, that patients with IC have an overactive fight or flight response, which upregulates the nervous system. This can make the body and mind react more strongly to stimuli, such as pain, inflammation, or stress: The same notes that used to be soothing elevator jazz now sound like they're coming from the front row of a Metallica concert.

Other evidence points to a bigger problem with the nervous system. Early studies have shown that patients with IC can have other symptoms relating to nervous system regulation, such as fainting and difficulty regulating blood pressure. Although it remains to be seen whether this is due to an underlying problem or is somehow caused by IC, nervous system upregulation is clearly an issue that exacerbates the symptoms of IC and must be addressed to treat the condition.

Pain Tolerance

Could patients with IC actually be worse at processing pain? Most patients would say no—they'd argue that their pain tolerance is high because they deal with a lot of pain on a daily basis. However, this raises an important distinction when it comes to discussing pain.

Pain is subjective and experienced differently by everyone. It is commonly—and studies show quite accurately—measured on a 10-point scale, with 0 being no pain at all and 10 being the worst pain imaginable. When people talk about a "high pain tolerance," they typically mean they function well considering the amount of pain they're in. This is very true for many IC patients, who courageously go about their daily activities in a substantial amount of pain.

Another important concept is "pain threshold." This is the point at which a given stimulus becomes painful. Imagine you're holding a hot beverage. It may feel pleasantly warm at a lower temperature; it might start getting uncomfortable if it's hotter; and finally it becomes burning hot to touch. The point at which it becomes painful is the pain threshold.

Some evidence indicates that patients with IC actually have a lowered threshold to pain, because of the upregulation of the nervous system. Stimuli that normally wouldn't be uncomfortable are reported as painful, and pain that would be relatively mild in someone else is translated as "excruciating" by the brain. For example, you'd feel a painful burn when a coffee mug was only lukewarm, but your friend could hold it comfortably. Is this the "reason" you have IC? No—but could this heightened sensitivity make you more susceptible to bladder ulcers or filling? To an inflamed bladder lining? To pelvic floor dysfunction? Almost certainly.

 Pain Tolerance vs. Threshold

Pain tolerance: "Even though I was in 6-out-of-10 pain, I still got up and made breakfast for my children before going to work."

Pain threshold: "I'm experiencing 6-out-of-10 pain when I pee, when someone who wasn't used to chronic pain might only be feeling a little discomfort with the same sensation."

"Many IC patients courageously go about their daily activities in a substantial amount of pain."

Estrogen's Role

Many women notice changes in their symptoms at different points during their cycles. Estrogen has been found to play a role in other chronic pain conditions, and one small study reported increased symptoms in IC patients when estrogen peaks in the week prior to menses (the onset of menstruation). Anecdotally, flares due to hormones are most likely during ovulation or in the week before menses, when estrogen levels are highest. Many women experience an easing of symptoms during periods when their estrogen levels are lowest. Some patients report an improvement in symptoms and reduced flares when they use oral contraceptives, which can stabilize estrogen levels throughout the cycle.

Pelvic Surgeries and the Risk for IC

In 2013, researchers from the University of Maryland published study results showing a correlation between pelvic surgery and IC. They noticed that patients were fifteen times more likely to have had a nonbladder pelvic surgery in the month prior to an IC diagnosis. If the surgery was a hysterectomy, the odds jumped to twenty-five times. This is a striking connection, and can't be dismissed as coincidence.

This information may provide important clues about IC, but it raises more questions than it answers. Do unrelated pelvic surgeries somehow cause IC? There is always trauma associated with a surgery, which draws inflammation to the affected region. The incision sites can scar as they heal and may become stuck to organs or other tissue in the pelvic region, causing dysfunction and tightness. If those scars (known as surgical adhesions) stick to the bladder, they might impede its ability to fill, putting additional strain and pressure on the organ.

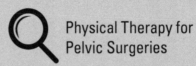

Physical Therapy for Pelvic Surgeries

Pelvic surgeries are often incredibly invasive and can have lingering effects on some of the most vital functions of the body, yet they are also the only major type of surgery where physical therapy (PT) isn't automatically suggested for patients. Postsurgical PT ensures scar tissue doesn't adhere, rebuilds strength, and restores normal function and range of motion after the operation.

Common pelvic surgeries include C-sections, hysterectomies, prostatectomies, and colorectal surgeries. Don't be afraid to ask about pelvic PT after these procedures. Even a few postsurgical visits can prevent many complications and set you up for a more complete recovery.

Another potential explanation is that interstitial cystitis may be a condition that underlies many other causes of pelvic pain, such as endometriosis and vulvodynia. In fact, researchers found that nearly 80 percent of patients with generalized pelvic pain may have undiagnosed interstitial cystitis. If the IC symptoms are masked by more pressing symptoms from a condition, such as endometriosis, you may not notice them until the source of the endometriosis pain (the uterus) has been removed. The increased chance of an IC diagnosis after an unrelated surgery may be because IC was the underlying reason for the pelvic pain that necessitated the surgery, and because the surgical trauma brings out the "classic" IC symptoms that lay dormant. Pain from interstitial cystitis can present in many different ways, and it is possible that doctors and patients are attributing IC pain to another organ or site, planning surgeries to correct or remove the perceived source of the pain—and only later realizing that interstitial cystitis was the root cause.

In any case—whether pelvic surgeries increase the risk for IC or IC is an underlying cause in other surgeries thought to be unrelated—be aware of this risk if you undergo pelvic surgery, and be ready to address IC symptoms if they crop up afterward. Physical therapy can be an important part of achieving a full recovery from pelvic surgeries, and it can also alleviate IC symptoms if they arise post-surgery.

Takeaways

- **There is no single, accepted cause of interstitial cystitis.** Patients can be hopeful because the pace of research is accelerating. But IC is probably the result of multiple causes, and we may never have a satisfactory and comprehensive answer to it.

- **There is a complex interplay between the bladder, pelvic floor, and the nervous system.** Regardless of the underlying cause(s), it is clear that IC entangles the bladder, pelvic floor, and nerves in a pattern of dysfunction. All areas must be addressed to manage IC successfully.

- **Don't get caught up in the unknown.** We don't need to have all the answers to diagnose and successfully treat interstitial cystitis. It's easy to get caught up in and distracted by everything we don't know about the condition, but remember that many other medical problems are also poorly understood. What really matters is how to address the symptoms of IC, and how to regain control of your health.

4

THE STRUGGLE FOR ANSWERS:

The Road to Diagnosis

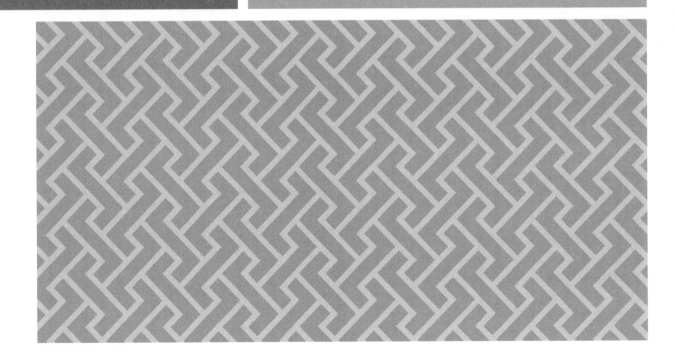

W hen we face medical challenges, we want the certainty that comes with a concrete diagnosis. Giving a name to the culprit gives us power over it, and reassures us that the medical community has a plan for handling the condition.

No one likes to hear "maybe" from their doctor. That's why it's frustrating that nearly every IC diagnosis begins with that very word. The American Urologic Association (AUA) says there are many problems with "misdiagnosis, under-diagnosis, and delayed diagnosis." And nearly every patient with IC that I've treated would confirm they've had problems in obtaining an initial diagnosis. The fact is that taking control of your health starts by navigating the treacherous path to an accurate IC diagnosis, and this chapter guides you there.

Diagnosing interstitial cystitis is difficult because it can only be identified when everything else has been ruled out. As noted before, there is no positive test for IC in which your exam results prove you have the condition. You can only be diagnosed by your symptoms and the lack of another explanation. To diagnose IC, a doctor must rule out a common urinary tract infection (UTI), as well as rare conditions, such as bladder cancer or bladder stones. In men, there is a great deal of confusion between chronic nonbacterial prostatitis and IC. Other conditions that present as potential explanations include an overactive bladder, general pelvic floor dysfunction, or sexually transmitted diseases.

The largest prevalence study in women was conducted by the nonprofit RAND Corporation and published in 2011. After contacting more than 130,000 households, the authors found that women with IC had seen an average of 3.5 doctors about their condition, but less than 10 percent had been correctly diagnosed with interstitial cystitis. Less than 50 percent had received any diagnosis at all—even an incorrect one!

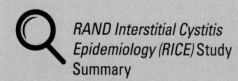

RAND Interstitial Cystitis Epidemiology (RICE) Study Summary

- 130,000 households interviewed
- 12 million people with IC
- Each patient had been seen by an average of 3.5 doctors
- *Only 9.7 percent were correctly diagnosed*

Medical Training and IC Diagnosis

The RICE study statistics may seem staggering, but remember the vast majority of doctors have not been trained in the modern definition of interstitial cystitis. The AUA only released their first guidelines for diagnosis and treatment in 2011, and textbooks need time to incorporate the latest research. That means it's nearly certain that your doctor was trained with outdated information about IC—if he or she learned much about the condition at all. Plus, with ongoing medical advancements, it's impossible for a single doctor to keep up with information in all specialties. Your primary-care doctor or an urgent-care clinic may never have diagnosed a patient with IC, and it's unlikely your doctor is focusing his or her continuing education on the condition.

Every doctor you visit entered the world of medicine because they wanted to make a difference for patients, and are doing their best to help. Occam's razor—the idea that the simplest explanation is the most likely solution—guides most doctors. Medical students are trained to approach diagnoses like this: "When you hear hoofbeats, think horses, not zebras." This reminds doctors to assume that the most common disease or condition is causing a patient's symptoms until proven otherwise. This is the logical approach, but if you are starting with faulty information—for example, that IC is uncommon— misdiagnosis can result. The best prevalence studies, which have indicated that more than twelve million Americans likely have this condition, were done only recently. So, when your doctor went through medical school, she probably learned that IC was an unlikely diagnosis. But the truth is that it's extremely common; IC is the horse, not the zebra.

Urinary Tract Infections and IC

Urinary tract infections (UTIs) are caused by bacteria that invade the urinary tract and bladder. Almost half of women will have at least one UTI in their lives. Chances of contracting a UTI increase with pregnancy, sexual activity, or any condition that may compromise the immune system. Both UTIs and IC can cause pain, urgency, and frequency, and, prior to an IC diagnosis, both doctor and patient often have difficulty believing the symptoms are not due to an infection—even after a urinalysis or urine culture comes back negative. Almost everyone begins their IC journey believing they have a simple UTI. To make things even more confusing, IC patients are more likely to have a history of UTIs—nearly one-third of patients diagnosed with interstitial cystitis also had a recently confirmed UTI. So, testing positive for a UTI doesn't necessarily rule out IC; sometimes the UTI is treated, but many of the symptoms still persist.

IC: A Doctor's Perspective

One of my IC patients is a family-care physician, and working with him was extremely interesting. He prides himself on being an excellent diagnostician— and, to his credit, he successfully diagnosed himself with interstitial cystitis.

From his perspective, most doctors want to address your problem with a procedure or medication they know and can control. They want something they can fix; it's where they feel their value lies. After all, it's human nature to light up with enthusiasm when we encounter a problem we're uniquely qualified to solve.

Treating IC or chronic pelvic pain is completely different. It's a journey, and there's no easy answer or quick fix. One reason to find a specialist, beyond education or qualifications, is that specialists *want to treat patients like you*. They have a passion for treating difficult, chronic conditions, and understand that it takes more than a simple procedure or prescription. They know the true value of a multidisciplinary team, and seek out other practitioners to be part of your solution. That's the kind of doctor you deserve.

For more information on finding the right doctor or specialist, see page 189.

A traditional urinary tract infection is relatively simple to detect and to treat. A bacterial infection is confirmed with a positive dipstick test and a positive urine culture. It will respond quickly to an appropriate prescription antibiotic, and should resolve within a few days. However, UTIs can sometimes be tricky and more difficult to diagnose or treat. The dipstick test may be negative or ambiguous (when it "kind of" changes colors). Or, the test in the doctor's office may be negative, but, after sending it out to culture, the more accurate lab testing uncovers the presence of a UTI. Treatment with antibiotics should resolve the symptoms, but, if the bacteria are resistant to antibiotics, the first round may not be effective. When you return to the doctor, the urinalysis will still test positive for bacteria, and a different antibiotic should be prescribed.

Then there's the "phantom UTI"—the dipstick test is negative, and the full culture is also negative (or isn't run at all). With your symptoms, it's still easiest to assume it's probably a UTI—after all, what else could it be?—so you end up with a prescription for antibiotics anyway. Of course, they won't be effective, and you'll be back in your doctor's office a week later.

As a patient, don't get stuck in the medical purgatory of assuming negative tests for UTIs are repeatedly incorrect. Some patients receive a negative test result for a UTI and then take a round of antibiotics "just to be safe." This can happen repeatedly—another negative test, a different type of antibiotic. Suddenly, six months have passed and you haven't explored any options beyond a possible UTI. As a general rule of thumb, if you've been experiencing UTI-like symptoms and the urine culture comes back negative and/or a round of antibiotics hasn't helped, your doctor should consider other possibilities. Your primary-care physician or an urgent-care doctor may not have experience with interstitial cystitis, and may continue treating phantom UTIs unless you find a specialist or suggest a different approach.

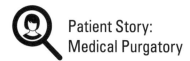

Patient Story: Medical Purgatory

Joanna came to see me reporting urinary urgency, frequency, and pelvic pain. When the symptoms began months before, her first thought was that she had a UTI, so she went to her primary-care physician.

On her first visit, the dipstick test was positive, so she went home with a course of antibiotics. When her symptoms didn't improve, she scheduled another appointment.

On the second visit, the dipstick test was positive again. But, this time, they sent the sample to the lab where more accurate testing showed no bacteria. Still, Joanna was given a prescription for a more powerful antibiotic. This time her symptoms eased over the next three to four weeks, but didn't go away completely. After a business trip, with long flights and days of extended sitting, her symptoms returned with a vengeance.

When she returned to her doctor the third time, he took her improvement as evidence the antibiotics were working, but just weren't strong enough to eliminate the infection. With no additional testing, she was given a third round of antibiotics.

This process spanned four months. During this time, Joanna had almost constant stomach problems due to the increasingly powerful antibiotics. The cycle of dysfunction, inflammation, and pain was escalated, until she could hardly sit without flaring her symptoms. While she may—or may not—have had a UTI at first, it soon became clear that there was more going on.

Initial Exam for IC

When the presence of IC is suspected, your examination should include a medical history, physical exam, and basic lab tests. You'll be asked about the history, location, and severity of any pelvic pain and about urinary symptoms, including urinary frequency and urgency. The history will also note whether you have any pain with sex, urination, ejaculation (for men), and whether it changes with your menstrual cycle (for women). Report any other symptoms you have in the pelvic region, even if you aren't sure they're related. Low back, hip, and tailbone pain can all be caused or influenced by the pelvic floor and IC. Tell your doctor whether anything seems to improve or exacerbate your symptoms. A full bladder, long periods of sitting, constipation, certain foods, and stress commonly influence IC symptoms.

If you suspect you may have IC, or have had frequent UTIs that have caused multiple visits to the doctor, you should keep a symptom diary that can help with diagnosis (see chapter 2). Take daily notes about your pain levels and locations and your urinary symptoms so you can share them with your doctor upon initial examination. Keep this symptom diary for at least a week prior to your doctor's appointment. Also make note of anything you experienced that was out of the ordinary—a particularly rich meal at a restaurant, a long drive, consumption of alcohol, anything especially stressful—because these events can have a marked effect on symptoms and can help your doctor understand what influences them.

This symptom diary is particularly important for women— unfortunately, women are more likely to be dismissed, or to have their testimony discounted, by a doctor. Studies have shown that women are more likely than men to be denied appropriate pain medication. But it's much more difficult for a doctor to dismiss a detailed symptom diary that spans at least a week than it is to ignore general complaints of pain.

Make the Most of Your Doctor's Appointment

Here's a brief list of what you should bring to your doctor's appointment to make the most of your limited time with your doctor—and to ensure your concerns are heard. (For more detailed descriptions of these categories, see page 191.)

- Written list detailing your worst 3 to 4 symptoms
- List of any other symptoms that you may notice
- Symptom diary
- Bladder diary
- Written timeline of symptoms and/or treatments
- Any previous testing results
- Easing/aggravating factors
- Medications you've tried or are currently taking

In addition to the symptom diary, it's also important to have filled out a bladder diary documenting your urinary habits and food and fluid intake. Having at least three consecutive days of a bladder diary can provide your doctor with valuable clues to help with diagnosis.

Instructions: In the first column, note everything you eat and drink over the course of the day. (Estimate how much you drink in ounces or cups.) Next, record each trip to the bathroom and how many seconds the stream lasted. Rate how urgently you needed to go (0 = not at all; 4 = you couldn't hold it any longer), and whether there was any incontinence. Finally, note what you were doing at the time—your physical position (sitting, standing, lying), where you were, and anything else that is relevant. At the end of each day, add up your total fluid intake, number of trips to the bathroom, and any notes on your overall activity (spent all day sitting in meetings, hiking, etc.).

SAMPLE BLADDER DIARY

DATE: _____

Time of day	Food/drink intake	Bathroom trip (X)	Seconds	Urge to go (0 to 4)	Leaks (Y/N)	Activity notes: What were you doing at the time?
6 to 7 a.m.	Bagel, herbal tea	X	15	2	N	Just woke up
		X	6	4	N	Sitting in uncomfortable kitchen chair
7 to 8 a.m.						
8 to 9 a.m.						
9 to 10 a.m.						
10 to 11 a.m.						
11 to 12 p.m.						
12 to 1 p.m.						
1 to 2 p.m.						
2 to 3 p.m.						

SAMPLE BLADDER DIARY *(continued)*

Time of day	Food/drink intake	Bathroom trip (X)	Seconds	Urge to go (0 to 4)	Leaks (Y/N)	Activity notes: What were you doing at the time?
3 to 4 p.m.						
4 to 5 p.m.						
5 to 6 p.m.						
6 to 7 p.m.						
7 to 8 p.m.						
8 to 9 p.m.						
9 to 10 p.m.						
10 to 11 p.m.						
Nighttime						
Total	Total fluid intake:	Total bathroom trips:			Total leaks:	Overall activity notes:

Age of Onset

The age at which a patient is diagnosed with IC is often substantially later than when symptoms first arise. Because it can take many years—and multiple doctors—to diagnose interstitial cystitis correctly, symptoms are usually present long before middle age. The 2011 *RICE* study (see summary on page 45), indicates the initial onset of symptoms is more likely to occur in a woman's twenties than her forties. Many case reports have found IC in women under the age of eighteen—though typically patients under eighteen are not evaluated in scientific studies. And many doctors, having read that IC diagnosis typically occurs around or after age forty, may disregard symptoms in younger patients. But in one study of medical students at the University of California, San Diego, researchers found at least 10 percent of women in the class had IC. The students' average age was twenty-six. This is further proof that IC can occur at any age, and may actually be more typical in younger patients.

Diagnosis in Men

The prevalence of interstitial cystitis in men is another area in which a persistent myth hinders proper diagnosis. It's been assumed that IC was primarily a women's condition: As recently as 2014, the AUA Guidelines report that the ratio of female to male patients may be as high as 10:1. However, that information is based on data decades old and substantially out of date.

The newest research challenges the long-held assumption that IC predominantly affects women. In the largest study to examine IC in men, also conducted by the RAND Corporation and published in 2013, the authors contacted nearly 5,000 households. Men were interviewed regarding the symptoms of interstitial cystitis, using the same criteria validated in their groundbreaking study of women. They found the prevalence of

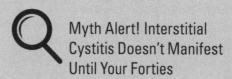

Myth Alert! Interstitial Cystitis Doesn't Manifest Until Your Forties

Fact: IC can be diagnosed at any age.

The general consensus on when IC typically occurs has been based on old and faulty data, making its diagnosis even more difficult. Many textbooks and guidelines report that the diagnosis is typically made when the patient is around forty years old. However, little evidence is ever cited to support this statistic. When the American Urology Association mentioned this in their guidelines about interstitial cystitis, the sole source they cited was a single study published in 2003. This study evaluated only twenty patients in a single county over a twenty-year span! Based on only sixteen women (diagnosed at age 44.5 years) and four men (diagnosed at age 71.5), urologists across the country may be hesitant to diagnose interstitial cystitis in younger patients. To make matters worse, for most of the duration of this study (conducted from 1976 to 1996), IC didn't even have a formal definition! It reports data from a tiny subset of patients, in a minuscule region, during an era in which many doctors thought IC was a psychiatric condition.

IC in men was much higher than had been assumed. Depending on the definition of IC, the authors found that between 1.9 and 4.2 percent of men have interstitial cystitis, which is very similar to the range of 2.7 to 6.5 percent they found in women. Instead of being a condition that almost exclusively affects women, the ratio of female to male patients may in fact be nearly equal. This has major implications for the diagnosis and treatment of IC, which may not be nearly as rare in men as doctors assume.

So why does the myth that women are substantially more likely to have IC persist? Older studies are unreliable because they used a lengthy and exhaustive list of symptoms to define IC. For example, to be considered IC, a cystoscopy had to show glomerulations (little red dots now thought to be completely irrelevant in IC diagnosis) spread throughout the bladder. The symptoms had to be present for at least nine months (only six weeks is required for a diagnosis today), and you couldn't be diagnosed if you'd had a UTI within the past three months (nearly one-third of IC patients have had a recent UTI). These were just a few of the eighteen different restrictions on the definition of IC—it's actually a miracle any cases were diagnosed at all!

Some retrospective studies review old case files to calculate the number of patients that have been diagnosed with the condition. But because doctors have been told that IC is rare in men, they are unlikely to diagnose it and lean instead toward male-centric conditions, such as chronic prostatitis. Then researchers tally those diagnoses and publish results that show men don't get IC, and the process repeats itself. This kind of circular reasoning is why population-based studies—in which a large number of random people are called and interviewed—are the gold standard in determining a condition's prevalence.

This is also why the recent *RICE* studies are so crucial to our understanding of the condition. Researchers examined a random segment of the population using the modern definition of IC. They also had the foresight to include chronic prostatitis questions to determine the overlap. Their estimate of 4.2 percent of men with IC is slightly lower than, but similar to, the rates in women.

Chronic Prostatitis and IC in Men

The diagnosis of IC in men is often muddled by another condition: chronic prostatitis/chronic pelvic pain syndrome (CP/CPPS). According to the American Urologic Association, CP/CPPS is a condition "characterized by pain in the perineum, suprapubic region, testicles, or tip of the penis often exacerbated by urination… Voiding symptoms, such as a sense of incomplete bladder emptying and urinary frequency, are also commonly reported." Sound familiar?

Many researchers believe that chronic prostatitis may actually be a manifestation of interstitial cystitis. The symptoms of suprapubic and perineum pain are classic IC symptoms, and the pelvic floor dysfunction that accompanies IC has been shown to cause testicular and penile pain. Previous studies have shown that more than half of men with IC have pain with ejaculation—another hallmark of chronic prostatitis. Population-based studies have shown that up to 90 percent of those with chronic prostatitis symptoms could be diagnosed with interstitial cystitis instead.

OVERLAP BETWEEN IC AND CHRONIC PROSTATITIS

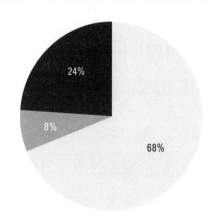

Interstitial cystitis only

Chronic prostatitis only

■ Both conditions

24%

8%

68%

Source: Suskind, A., S. Berry, B. Ewing, et al. "The Prevalence and Overlap of Interstitial Cystitis/Bladder Pain Syndrome and Chronic Prostatitis/Chronic Pelvic Pain Syndrome in Men: Results of the RAND Interstitial Cystitis Epidemiology (RICE) Male Study," *The Journal of Urology* 189, no.1 (January 2013): 141-45.

SYMPTOM COMPARISON BETWEEN INTERSTITIAL CYSTITIS IN MEN AND CHRONIC PROSTATITIS

	Interstitial cystitis in men	Chronic prostatitis
Pain	• suprapubic • bladder • testicular • perineal	• suprapubic • bladder • testicular • perineal • penile
Urinary	• frequency • hesitancy • incomplete voiding • urgency	• frequency • hesitancy • incomplete voiding
Diet	90 percent affected	47 percent affected
Diagnosis	by exclusion	by exclusion
Potassium sensitivity in bladder	78 percent	84 percent
Treatment	• no consistent medication • physical therapy • diet • lifestyle	• no consistent medication • physical therapy • diet • lifestyle

"When it comes to male urinary symptoms, urologists tend to blame the prostate, which can result in prostate cancer scares and steer male patients away from an IC diagnosis."

Because of the similarities between these conditions, some researchers have proposed the use of an umbrella term of Urologic Chronic Pelvic Pain Syndrome (UCPPS) to describe both IC and chronic prostatitis, where IC and CP would be subtypes of the broader category.

Regardless of whether IC and CP are the same condition, two related conditions, or totally independent of one another, the practical implications for male patients are clear. Both IC and CP are characterized by pelvic floor dysfunction, which causes pain, sexual dysfunction, and urinary symptoms. The AUA Guidelines note that treatment for IC has been shown to help chronic prostatitis patients: The benefits of oral medication, physical therapy, stretching, changes in diet, and lifestyle changes are shared between IC and CP. The majority of those diagnosed with CP—even if it continues to be listed as a separate condition—may also have IC, and can benefit from the IC treatments outlined in this book, especially those that address pelvic floor dysfunction and pelvic floor physical therapy.

■ *Stigma of IC Symptoms in Men*

Although women are often at risk for having their symptoms dismissed as "hysteria" or a psychiatric condition, men's symptoms also may be discounted by doctors. When younger men report IC symptoms, the first instinct of many doctors is to blame drugs or an STD. Male patients may believe that their urinary symptoms are just an ordinary part of aging. When it comes to male urinary symptoms, urologists tend to blame the prostate, which can result in prostate cancer scares and steer male patients away from an IC diagnosis.

Medical Procedures and Diagnosis

The medical community has recently made a major shift in thinking regarding the use of medical procedures for diagnosing interstitial cystitis. In the past, a painful and expensive barrage of medical procedures was standard prior to an IC diagnosis. Current protocols now state that these medical procedures, such as cystoscopies and urodynamics, are unnecessary for diagnosing simple cases of IC but can aid in diagnosing the most complex cases. These tests can only be used to exclude other possibilities—in the same way that a urinalysis can rule out a UTI—not to diagnose IC. They can give important information but are not required for a diagnosis, and some procedures that used to be routine have been shown to be completely unnecessary. Following are the most common medical procedures conducted in conjunction with a suspected IC diagnosis.

Don't ever be afraid to ask your doctor why a specific procedure or test is conducted. Since the guidelines for treatment from the American Urologic Society were only first published in 2011, many doctors may not yet be familiar with the most recent recommendations. Your doctor should be able to express clearly to you the purpose of the test, what she hopes to learn from it, and how that information will guide your treatment. The AUA Guidelines state that these medical procedures should only be conducted if they have the potential to alter the treatment approach or to rule out other conditions that might be responsible for the symptoms.

Cystoscopy

A cystoscopy is a procedure in which a small camera on a flexible cable is inserted through the urethra to view of the inside of the bladder. In cases of suspected interstitial cystitis, the cystoscopy is usually conducted to find damage in the bladder lining and rule out bladder cancer as a possible cause of the symptoms. Because bladder cancer can cause some of the same symptoms, it is often ruled out before a formal diagnosis of interstitial cystitis is given. However, bladder cancer is relatively rare—you are seven to twenty times more likely to have IC than cancer. A cystoscopy can also find Hunner's lesions in a small percentage of IC patients and can cauterize these lesions if they exist.

This procedure is typically performed under local anesthesia but can be very uncomfortable for patients, especially when the bladder and urethra are already irritated, so some IC patients request a "twilight" anesthesia to minimize the pain and discomfort. You should be prepared for a flare in symptoms following a cystoscopy. Although it's not required, almost all doctors will do a cystoscopy when bladder pain is involved.

What doctors should *not* be seeking during a cystoscopy are glomerulations—small areas of broken blood vessels that show up as little red dots on the camera. Historically, these red dots were thought to indicate IC, but recent research has shown they carry almost no predictive value. Almost 50 percent of people *without* IC symptoms have these glomerulations, and up to one-third of IC patients won't have any glomerulations at

all. Even the majority of patients with overactive bladder have visible glomerulations during a cystoscopy. These little broken blood vessels can be completely asymptomatic; they can be the result of the procedure itself, or completely unrelated to interstitial cystitis.

Urodynamics

Urodynamic evaluation is designed to test how the bladder and urethra are functioning. This series of tests, usually performed by a urologist or urogynecologist, can determine how rapidly the bladder empties, how much residual urine remains in the bladder, and the pressure in the urethra.

The procedure for urodynamics is uncomfortable and difficult. It involves sitting on a glorified toilet with a catheter in your urethra, an electrode in your vagina (for women), and external electrodes placed around your perineum and anal sphincter. Your bladder is artificially filled and your muscle contractions are measured to see when your bladder first begins to spasm. The system can measure whether there is any leakage (incontinence) and how full the bladder is when you have your first urge to urinate, when pain occurs, and the overall capacity of the bladder. The most common reason for this procedure is to diagnose overactive bladder, which is not typically accompanied by pain. The presence of pelvic pain—suprapubic, urethral, bladder, or elsewhere—indicates interstitial cystitis, and urodynamic evaluation is often unnecessary.

Unless your doctor has a very compelling reason to perform a urodynamic evaluation, this procedure rarely adds value to IC diagnosis or treatment. It really shouldn't be performed unless you see no improvement with multiple IC treatments and your doctor is concerned there may be another condition to address.

Potassium Sensitivity Test

A painful and outdated procedure, the potassium sensitivity test is no longer recommended to diagnose interstitial cystitis. In this evaluation, a solution of potassium is instilled into the bladder and the level of pain and urinary urgency are compared against a solution of plain saline. This test has been shown to result in false positives, particularly when a bacterial infection is present, and fails to detect IC in at least 20 percent of patients. The American Urologic Association has determined this test is unnecessary, extremely painful, and should not be performed in suspected IC patients.

Phenotyping

Phenotyping attempts to divide IC patients into subgroups based on their symptoms. Its ultimate goal is to determine which kind of treatment will be most successful for an individual patient, customizing treatment and avoiding the current trial-and-error approach. This area of research holds promise for patients, but requires significantly more study before it can have a practical benefit for those diagnosed with IC.

Methods of Phenotyping

1949 Method: Divides patients into Grade 1, 2, or 3, based on evidence of bladder damage on cystoscopy.

Painful Bladder Syndrome versus IC: Makes the common distinction between patients with evidence of bladder damage and those without. Patients without Hunner's lesions are diagnosed with Painful Bladder Syndrome, while the term IC is reserved for those with evidence of bladder wounds.

UPOINT System: Classifies patients by predominating symptoms, and it's currently the focus of a lot of research. The symptom categories used are urinary, psychosocial, organ-specific, infection, neurologic, and tenderness. Many patients fall into several categories, making a firm phenotype difficult—although, with additional research, it may be possible to "cluster" patients into groups that experience two or more symptom types.

Body Pain Phenotypes: Categorizes patients by the number of pain sites on the body in addition to IC. Though it's possible simply to have IC symptoms, some patients also experience pain in other areas of the body. Some researchers who support this method of phenotyping believe untreated symptoms of interstitial cystitis can lead to pain in other locations.

Currently, patients are often divided into different subgroups based on how they respond to different treatments. However, the goal of phenotyping is to determine the sorts of treatments to which patients will respond well, and to guide them into that treatment course: It defeats the purpose if patients must try different types of treatments to determine their phenotypes. Given how complicated the condition is many patients also cross over into multiple potential categories. So, to be a helpful tool for patients, better criteria need to be discovered to place patients into categories at an earlier stage.

It is also unclear whether treatments will be more successful with one phenotype than another. Even if researchers agree on a universal system of phenotyping, it does no practical good unless the treatment plan is different for each phenotype. Clinical trials would have to be repeated, with the patients divided into these phenotypes, to see whether there is any difference in the way patients respond to treatment. Until we have both a simple, accepted method of phenotyping and evidence that these different phenotypes respond differently to treatment, patients will not see a practical benefit from phenotyping.

Another major challenge with phenotyping is the length of time it takes for a patient to receive a correct diagnosis of interstitial cystitis. The benefit of phenotyping is based on being able to divide patients into discrete subgroups, but if IC is left untreated, it tends to expand into different categories. Most patients who have struggled with IC for years before receiving a proper diagnosis and treatment fall under multiple categories. That's why it's vital to diagnose the condition early—specifically in the first six months—before patients fall into the chronic pain cycle, which further complicates the diagnosis.

Takeaways

- **Interstitial cystitis is chronically under-diagnosed.** Fewer than 10 percent of patients believed to have the condition have received a formal diagnosis. Nearly ten million people are living, undiagnosed, with the symptoms of IC.

- **The underdiagnosis of IC is partially due to persistent myths.** Many doctors still believe interstitial cystitis is a rare condition, when in fact it affects more than twelve million Americans. Those unfamiliar with IC may believe it doesn't typically strike until middle age, while the latest research shows it's actually more likely to manifest in the patient's twenties. IC is still considered a problem that mainly affects women, even though nearly as many men may have the condition. Bladder lesions, glomerulations, cystoscopies, and urodynamics aren't necessary to diagnose IC. Don't fall victim to these myths as you navigate your diagnosis.

- **Don't stop seeking an explanation.** When it comes to IC symptoms, the first suspect is a urinary tract infection. If you aren't careful you could waste months, or even years, trying to eradicate a UTI that doesn't exist. If your current doctor is unable or unwilling to consider a diagnosis other than a bacterial infection for your symptoms, you may need to find a specialist. The sooner you receive an accurate IC diagnosis the sooner you can start on your healing journey.

5

THE PELVIC FLOOR CONNECTION:

It's Not Just Your Bladder

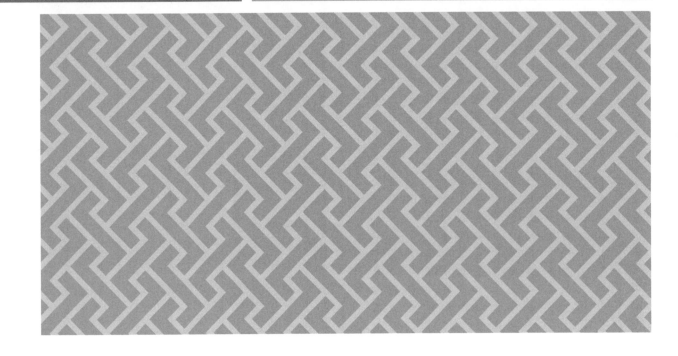

Most doctors—and many patients—think of IC primarily as a bladder condition. After all, the pain often appears to emanate from it, and the urinary urgency and frequency are certainly connected to the bladder and urethra. But the bladder isn't the whole story. Drugs have been developed to protect the bladder, but are ineffective in the majority of patients. And, in many cases of IC, there is no evidence of bladder damage—even under the most detailed inspection, the bladder often appears completely normal. The acidity and composition of urine haven't been shown to have any influence on symptoms, either. In extreme cases, the entire bladder is surgically removed—and yet the pain of IC often persists. So, if the bladder isn't solely responsible for IC symptoms, what's the missing piece?

The fact is that the bladder doesn't exist in isolation. It's intricately connected with all the muscles, ligaments, and tissue that surround the organ, collectively known as the pelvic floor. These muscles support the bladder and control its functions. They're why you're able to decide when to go to the bathroom and when to hold it, squeezing all day long to prevent urine from leaking out and then relaxing so you can urinate when you want to. And, every symptom of interstitial cystitis—suprapubic pain, urinary urgency and frequency, nocturia, low back pain, incontinence, and the rest—can be caused by dysfunction in the pelvic floor.

This is incredibly important. Your symptoms may be coming from your bladder, your pelvic floor, or—most likely—a combination of the two. Problems in your pelvic floor irritate the bladder, and vice versa. Strain and overuse of the bladder cause dysfunction in the pelvic floor. And the pelvic floor is so complex and interconnected that something that starts as a small problem can quickly spread and engulf the entire system. You will need to address both the pelvic floor and the bladder to manage IC successfully.

Researchers have reported that 70 to 85 percent of patients with IC have pelvic floor muscles that are too tight—a condition known as a hypertonic pelvic floor. This leads to the presence of trigger points or little muscle spasms in the pelvis, just as a tight back can cause muscle knots and soreness. Those figures may even underreport the number of IC patients with pelvic floor dysfunction; nearly every patient who comes in for treatment with an IC diagnosis has at least some pelvic floor involvement in symptoms.

Most patients miss this critical piece of the IC puzzle because doctors tend to focus exclusively on the bladder. The first specialist most patients see is usually a urologist or urogynecologist, who specializes in the bladder and urinary tract. Doctors have even told my patients they "don't believe in pelvic floor muscle spasm," which is like saying you don't believe in headaches caused by neck tension. Medical treatments that address the bladder are an important component of a holistic treatment plan, but true recovery can't take place without addressing the pelvic floor.

Before we go any further, here's a friendly warning: This is probably the most scientifically complex chapter of the book because the pelvic floor has a complicated anatomy and structure. Medical jargon is kept to a minimum, but some terminology is necessary to explain the pelvic floor muscles and how they relate to interstitial cystitis. So, use this chapter as a reference as you go through the rest of the book. Feel free to flip back and forth to review. Don't worry if you feel a bit overwhelmed at first. After a few months of self-treatment and physical therapy, most patients know the pelvic floor better than their doctors do.

"A healthy pelvic floor can improve posture, enhance athletic performance, help with balance, and leave you feeling more energetic."

What Is a Trigger Point?

A trigger point is a tender area or knot within a muscle or connective tissue that causes musculoskeletal pain. It is often highly irritable when touched, but can also cause referred pain that radiates into other areas of the body, causing muscles to stiffen and resulting in dysfunction. In IC, trigger points can even reproduce urinary urgency and the burning sensation in the urethra with urination. Eliminating these trigger points is a major component of a holistic treatment plan.

The Pelvic Floor

The pelvic floor isn't just a clever name; it's literally the floor of your pelvis. Improving the pelvic floor can eliminate pain that runs down to the feet or up to the back. A healthy pelvic floor can improve posture, enhance athletic performance, help with balance, and leave you feeling more energetic. It affects, directly or indirectly, almost every aspect of our lives. To put it simply, the pelvic floor is a big deal.

What Is the Pelvic Floor?

Imagine your chest and abdomen as a big canister, with your abdominal muscles in the front and your back muscles in the back. The ribs wrap around your chest, providing it with structure and support. The top half of that canister is filled with the heart and lungs, and is sealed off by the diaphragm at the bottom of your lungs. The bottom half—your abdomen—contains most of the rest of your organs: your stomach, liver, kidneys, intestines, and bladder are all squeezed into this tiny space. The bottom of the canister, supporting those vital organs, is the pelvic floor. Your intestines, bladder, uterus (in women), prostate (in men), and rectum are all resting in this natural hammock slung between the pelvic bones. The pelvic floor is a gatekeeper: The only way anything gets out of your body through your bladder or intestines is through holes in your pelvic floor. There are three in women (urethra, vagina, and rectum) and two in men (urethra and rectum).

Every muscle of the pelvic floor is connected, either directly or indirectly, to the tailbone (coccyx). When the pelvic floor muscles tighten, they flex your coccyx like they would a tail. In fact, many evolutionary biologists believe the muscles of the pelvic floor originally evolved to control the tails of our distant primate ancestors. If you can imagine all the cool things a monkey can do with its tail, you'll probably be amazed to realize you possess all the same muscles.

From the tailbone, these muscles stretch out and attach at different points on the "bony pelvis." The bony pelvis consists of the hip bones, sit bones, tailbone, and lower back. These bones are also connected to all major muscles in the region, including the inner thigh muscles, quads (in the front of your thigh), hamstrings (down the back of your thigh), gluteal muscles (the buttocks), abdominal muscles, and lower back. Because so many different muscles attach to it, the pelvis can be affected by tightness or weakness in any of them, which can then cause problems within the pelvic floor. The reverse is also true: Dysfunction within the pelvis can cause pain in the lower back, hips, or thighs. With its crossroads location, the pelvic floor affects both your upper and lower body.

What Does the Pelvic Floor Do?

First, the pelvic floor is **sphincteric**. Its muscles provide the physical closure to the bodily openings in the pelvis. It wraps around the urethra, the vaginal opening (in women), and the anal opening. Even "at rest," the pelvic floor is still responsible for holding these openings shut. It can also deliberately tighten to close those openings as you frantically search for a bathroom. If this function is compromised waste products can leak out, resulting in urinary or fecal incontinence.

The pelvic floor must release and stay relaxed to void completely. If it's unable to loosen enough, it can be a cause of urinary retention, in which the bladder cannot empty completely. We tend to think of urinary symptoms in conjunction with IC, but pelvic floor dysfunction can also contribute to diarrhea, gas, bloating, constipation, and abdominal pain related to the intestines and rectum.

Second, the pelvic floor is **supportive**. It physically supports and upholds all the organs in your pelvic cavity. Strung across your bony pelvis and attaching to the tailbone, you can think of it as a hammock for the bladder, vagina, uterus, prostate, and rectum. It's important to keep these organs in their proper places; if this function is compromised, the pelvic organs can slip and, in the worst cases, actually begin to slide down through the vagina or rectal openings in what is known as a pelvic organ prolapse. If these pelvic organs aren't in place and properly supported, they can't do their jobs correctly.

Third, the pelvic floor is **stabilizing**. It provides support for your lower back and stability for your pelvis. It's only supposed to act as a secondary source of support, with your lower back and abdominal muscles bearing the brunt of stabilization. However, with up to 80 percent of people having lower back problems, the pelvic floor is often forced to come to the rescue, aiding the back and abdominal muscles in supporting your spine and pelvis. This puts more strain on the pelvic floor than it was designed to carry, and can be another contributing factor to pelvic floor dysfunction.

Finally, the pelvic floor is **sexual**. In both genders, muscles of the pelvic floor are responsible for sexual arousal, functioning, and orgasm.

In women, the pelvic floor must expand to allow penetration of the vagina. These muscles also assist in positioning the clitoris against the pubic bone to provide additional stimulation and aid in female orgasm. In men, the pelvic floor helps maintain erections and brings about ejaculation during orgasm.

The pelvic floor plays an important part in the complex mechanism of sexual pleasure and function: If these muscles don't function correctly, women can have pain with entry and intercourse, and men may experience erectile dysfunction, groin pain, and pain following ejaculation.

How Does the Pelvic Floor Do All This?

All of the previous may seem like an impossible combination of tasks for such a small (and often-overlooked) set of muscles to accomplish. How do they manage it? These muscles have several important characteristics that help them meet all the responsibilities of the pelvic floor, and understanding these characteristics can also be important for knowing how to restore normal function to a distressed pelvic floor.

The pelvic floor muscles are voluntary, meaning you have direct control over them and can decide when to engage them. This contrasts with the smooth muscles of the organs, which are run automatically by the body and over which we have no conscious control (which is a good thing, because you wouldn't want a moment of distraction to stop your heart from beating!). However, the pelvic floor muscles are active all the time. They

have to be working to support your organs, to keep you standing (or sitting), and to prevent urine from leaking out. You may have voluntary control over these muscles, but that doesn't mean you can engage each muscle individually, in the same way that many people can't wiggle their ears or arch a single eyebrow at a time. However, you can control whether the pelvic floor relaxes or tightens, and you have direct, conscious input on many of the important functions of the pelvic floor.

The other important feature of these muscles is they include both fast-twitch and slow-twitch muscle fibers, so they can fulfill diverse roles. Fast-twitch muscles are responsible for your body's rapid, powerful movements: Sprinting, jumping, or any other explosive action relies on fast-twitch fibers. They contract rapidly, but speed comes at a price: These muscles burn through their fuel swiftly and quickly become exhausted. Slow-twitch muscle fibers, on the other hand, are associated with endurance. For instance, nearly 80 percent of the muscle fibers in marathon runners are slow-twitch. They are much more efficient, and can work for long periods of time without tiring.

Your pelvic floor is made up of about 70 percent slow-twitch and 30 percent fast-twitch muscle fibers, which allow it to do widely different things. The slow-twitch muscles are great at stabilizing the body and the pelvis. They are engaged nearly all the time, supporting the pelvic organs and transferring energy back and forth from your upper and lower body. The fast-twitch muscles handle the rapid, powerful jobs assigned to the pelvic floor. They release to allow waste to leave the body, and are involved in sexual arousal and orgasm. By combining these two types of muscle fibers within the same structure, the pelvic floor is able to accomplish all the necessary tasks.

Anatomy of the Pelvic Floor

To understand why pelvic floor dysfunction occurs and how to restore normal function, consider the anatomy of the pelvic floor and bladder (see illustration below and on page 65). A few muscles are extremely important in the urinary symptoms of the pelvic floor, and are probably causing at least some of the urgency, urethral pain, and burning you thought were coming from your bladder. Other muscles are more likely to produce the suprapubic or pelvic pain that's a hallmark of IC. Still others cause intestinal problems, pain with sex, lower back pain, or groin pain. Knowing the anatomy of the pelvic floor and the kinds of problems caused by each muscle lets you tailor your treatment and ensures the best possible care.

FEMALE PELVIC FLOOR ANATOMY

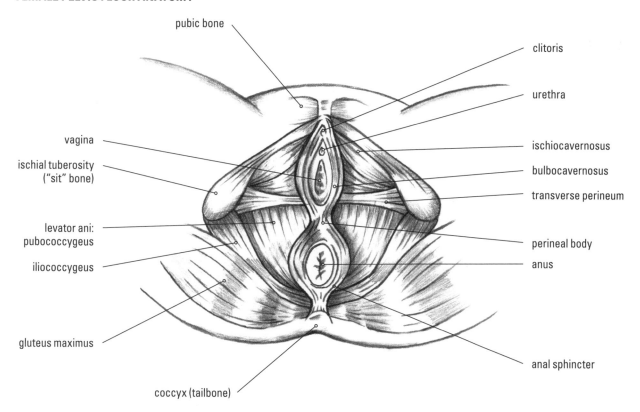

pubic bone

clitoris

urethra

vagina

ischiocavernosus

ischial tuberosity ("sit" bone)

bulbocavernosus

transverse perineum

levator ani: pubococcygeus

perineal body

iliococcygeus

anus

gluteus maximus

anal sphincter

coccyx (tailbone)

In this image, you can see how the pelvic floor muscles wrap around the urethra, vagina, and rectum. The muscles in the top half of this diagram—known as the urogenital triangle—are common culprits in bladder pain, urethral pain, and urinary urgency, while muscles in the bottom half are often responsible for pain with sex, low back pain, and hip pain.

MALE PELVIC FLOOR ANATOMY

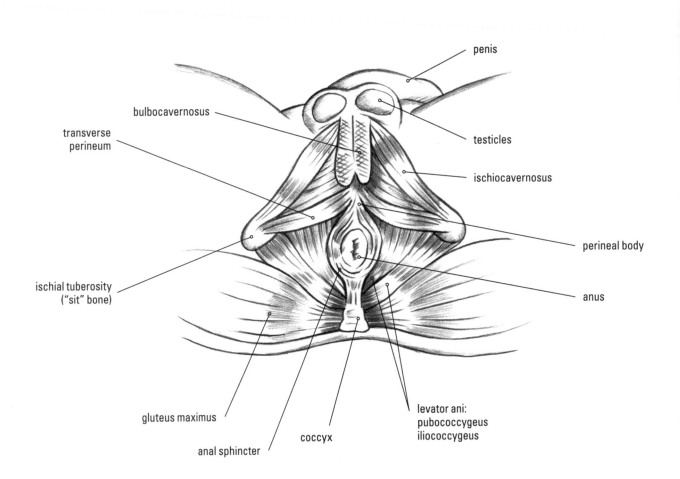

This view allows you to see both the superficial and deeper layers of the pelvic floor muscles.
The muscles of the pelvic floor wrap around the base of the penis and rectum, stretching from the pubic
bone to the tailbone, and trigger points in these muscles can create any of the symptoms of IC.

SIDE VIEW OF FEMALE PELVIS

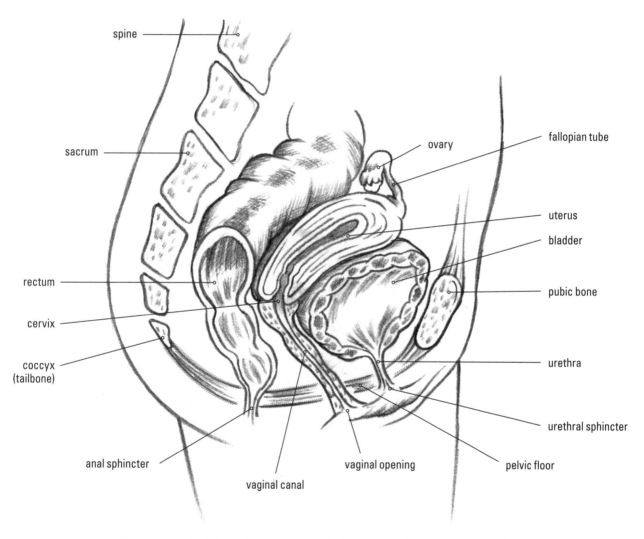

spine

sacrum

rectum

cervix

coccyx
(tailbone)

anal sphincter

vaginal canal

vaginal opening

ovary

fallopian tube

uterus

bladder

pubic bone

urethra

urethral sphincter

pelvic floor

Note the orientation of the female organs and their relationship to the bladder. Also notice the muscles
of the pelvic floor, stretching from the pubic bone to the tailbone. It's easy to see in this view how tightness
or trigger points in the pelvic floor muscles can affect the bladder, urethra, vagina, and rectum.

SIDE VIEW OF MALE PELVIS

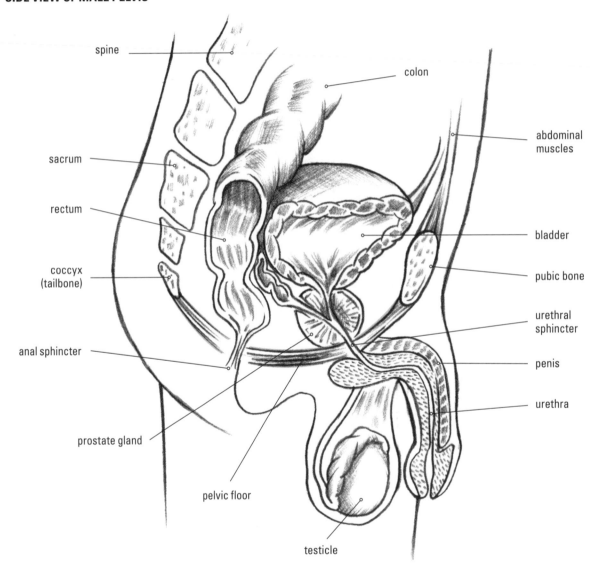

spine

colon

abdominal
muscles

sacrum

rectum

bladder

coccyx
(tailbone)

pubic bone

urethral
sphincter

anal sphincter

penis

urethra

prostate gland

pelvic floor

testicle

In this view, note how the urethra leaves the bladder and runs through the prostate before exiting the body through the pelvic floor. You can see how it may be difficult to determine whether the prostate (chronic prostatitis) or bladder (interstitial cystitis) is responsible for symptoms.

Ischiocavernosus

One of two muscles primarily responsible for bladder control, the "ischio" is often very tight and tender in IC patients (see pages 63 and 64). When trigger points develop here, they often manifest as urethral pain or burning. The ischiocavernosus is also often responsible for labial pain in women or pain deep in the groin for men, both of which can accompany IC.

Bulbocavernosus

The "bulbo" is another important muscle for people with interstitial cystitis (see pages 63 and 64). Along with the ischio, it's responsible for bladder control and is often very tight because of the urinary symptoms of IC. Trigger points here often reproduce the urethral pain and urinary symptoms of IC.

Urethral Sphincter

The urethral sphincter consists of two muscles that act as the bladder's gatekeepers (see pages 65 and 66). They are constantly engaged, preventing urine from escaping through the urethra: You deliberately tighten these muscles when you're actively squeezing to "hold it in," and you consciously release them when you're ready to use the restroom. When they have trigger points, they cause the urgent need to urinate that we associate with interstitial cystitis, or, alternatively, burning pain in the urethra. Many patients report this as a stinging sensation that occurs during urination or after it.

Superficial Transverse Perineum

The transverse perineum stretches across the pelvic floor, from sit bone to sit bone. It covers the area between the genitals and the anus (see pages 63 and 64). Problems here often manifest as pain or increased symptoms with sitting, and result in very tight hamstrings and inner thigh muscles. Feeling the transverse perineum is one of the best ways to assess your own pelvic floor without having to venture internally. Gently press on the perineum; it should feel spongy, and there shouldn't be any discomfort. But this area is often tender or uncomfortable to the touch when pelvic floor dysfunction is present.

Levator Ani

The levator ani is a series of muscles that we group together for the sake of convenience (see pages 63 and 64). Like all pelvic floor muscles, they attach to the coccyx and can actually move the tailbone. One of their primary functions is to help empty the bowels, which is one reason that problems with bowel movements—either constipation or diarrhea—can accompany pelvic floor dysfunction. Pressing on trigger points within the levator ani can recreate the feeling of needing to go to the bathroom. This muscle is one of the largest in the pelvic floor, and can also cause a lot of orthopedic pain: Hip, groin, buttock, or back pain often originates here.

Coccygeus

The primary responsibility of the coccygeus is to stabilize the tailbone (see page 68). Trigger points here often reproduce lower back and tailbone pain.

Piriformis and Obturator Internus

While these muscles aren't technically part of the pelvic floor, they share a close proximity, and can foster problems in the area (see page 68). A part of the gluteal and hip muscles, they're responsible for hip rotation and stabilization. The pudendal nerve, the major nerve that's responsible for most of the pelvic floor, runs close to both of these muscles. If they are tight or inflamed, they can put pressure on the pudendal nerve, which, in turn, can have wide-ranging consequences for the pelvic floor. When irritated, the pudendal nerve can cause any or all pelvic symptoms, including urinary symptoms and pain anywhere in the pelvic floor, sit bones, and gluteal fold.

TOP VIEW OF FEMALE PELVIC FLOOR

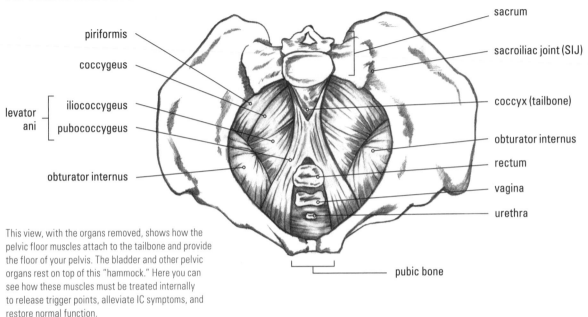

This view, with the organs removed, shows how the pelvic floor muscles attach to the tailbone and provide the floor of your pelvis. The bladder and other pelvic organs rest on top of this "hammock." Here you can see how these muscles must be treated internally to release trigger points, alleviate IC symptoms, and restore normal function.

Understanding the Bladder and Urinary System

The urinary system removes excess fluid and assorted waste from the body. The system starts with the kidneys, perhaps the hardest-working organs in the body. They filter the blood, siphoning off unnecessary fluid and removing waste from the bloodstream. The kidneys process your entire allowance of blood (about five quarts, 4.7 to 5 L) every hour, sorting through more than 120 quarts (114 L) of blood to distill about one to two quarts (946 ml to 1.9 L) of urine daily.

Once the urine is siphoned out by the kidneys, it makes its way to the bladder through the ureters (see pages 65 and 66). When empty, the bladder is like a deflated balloon, folded down on itself to the size and shape of a small pear. It sits behind your pubic bone, and it's hollow and muscular. It expands as it fills, and becomes spherical in shape as the fluid enters. The bladder's maximum capacity is two cups (475 ml), or almost exactly the amount of a small water bottle. Urine can be stored in the bladder for up to five hours before it is discharged.

The bladder is made up of smooth muscle (detrusor) that creates the structure of the bladder, which is protected from contact with the urine inside by the bladder lining (epithelium). The flexibility of the detrusor muscle is what allows the bladder to swell and contract as it fills and empties. Urine leaves the bladder through the urethra, which exits the body.

Keeping the urine inside the bladder is obviously an important task, and it's accomplished using two mechanisms. The first is an internal sphincter, made of the same muscle as the bladder, which naturally prevents urine from escaping. The pelvic floor is the ultimate gatekeeper. It is controlled voluntarily, so when you're rushing to find a bathroom, your pelvic floor holds back the tide until you're in position: It requires conscious permission to relax so you can void.

Urinary Tract Infections — Men and Women

One interesting anatomical difference between men and women in this region is the length of the urethra (see pages 65 and 66). In women, with the opening so close to the bladder, the urethra is quite short: In men, the urethra extends through the prostate and the length of the penis, so it's about five times longer. This is why women are so much more likely to have urinary tract infections than men. Due to proximity, it's much easier for foreign bacteria to navigate a woman's urethra and reach her bladder. With men, the additional length of the urethra makes it nearly impossible for the bacteria to "swim upstream" far enough to reach the bladder and cause an infection.

Normal Voiding

When the urinary system works normally, the brain is first informed that the bladder is filling when it's about one-quarter full. The stretching of the bladder triggers a signal that is sent to the brain: Specifically, the message is relayed to the frontal cortex, which is responsible for decision-making and strategic planning. This is the point at which you start consciously assessing your options: Where is the nearest bathroom? Is it clean? Would my friend think it rude if I interrupted his story in the middle to rush off and find it?

This system is designed to allow plenty of options. If a bathroom isn't available or convenient, you simply don't allow your pelvic floor to relax and release urine. You've been warned early, and your bladder has plenty of capacity, so you can push off the urge. As the bladder continues to fill, it will give you increasingly urgent warnings that get harder to ignore. Finally, when you have found a restroom, you give the pelvic floor permission to open the floodgates. The bladder contracts, "squeezing in" on itself until no urine remains. As it folds back down, it sends back the signal of relief to the brain. With interstitial cystitis, this complex system doesn't work properly.

■ Nervous System Upregulation

So how does such a normally reliable urinary system—designed to give you plenty of gentle forewarning about the need to urinate—go haywire when IC is involved? First, nervous system upregulation certainly plays a role. As we discussed earlier, nerves can become accustomed to being overused, and become more and more sensitive. In terms of the bladder, this means they're sending that first urge to use the bathroom a lot sooner than they should. Instead of getting your initial notice at one-quarter full, the bladder is sending the warning when there's only a fraction of that amount present—maybe just a few minutes after you last went. Then, each subsequent warning is more powerful, so you're receiving the signal normally associated with a bladder that's about to burst when it's only a quarter full instead. This is a cause of the frequent, but short, urinations that many people with interstitial cystitis experience.

■ *Interstitial Cystitis and Pelvic Floor Dysfunction*

The other problem is traced back to the tight, overworked pelvic floor. Its job is to prevent urine from escaping, so when you constantly feel the urge to use the bathroom and actively have to hold it in, your pelvic floor is working overtime—all day long.

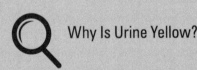

Why Is Urine Yellow?

The yellow color of urine and the brown color of feces actually come from the same source. Bilirubin is a component of bile (the gastric juice that helps digest fats) that breaks down into these different pigments. When it stays in the intestinal tract, this pigment remains brown and colors the feces. But when it is absorbed into the bloodstream and then processed through the kidneys, it's transformed into a yellow pigment that gives urine its distinctive color. The actual color of the final product changes depending on how diluted it is—the more water you drink, the lighter the color of your urine.

Just like any muscle in the body, being overworked can lead to problems. The muscles tighten and knots form in them, preventing them from stretching correctly to do their jobs. They become sore and tender. Some muscles become stronger than their neighbors through overuse, unbalancing the entire region. Worse, these muscles connect throughout the pelvic floor, so the damage isn't usually contained to just a single muscle. They all connect to the tailbone, so when one muscle puts extra stress on the coccyx, all the other muscles have to fire harder to keep the pelvic floor structure in place: That's why dysfunction in one muscle can throw the entire pelvic floor out of whack.

Trigger points in these pelvic floor muscles recreate the urgent need to urinate—but the tight muscles also make it difficult to urinate once you're in the bathroom. This is why many patients experience the paradox of an overwhelming urge to urinate, and then have difficulty actually starting a stream. And these tight muscles can make it difficult to empty the bladder fully, prompting the feeling that it's never quite empty, so the bladder doesn't send that relief signal back to the brain.

These knots also refer pain to different areas throughout the pelvic floor. They irritate the nerves and pelvic floor and send pain radiating throughout the region. Dysfunction in some muscles can specifically reproduce the urgency of urination experienced in IC, while others can be responsible for suprapubic pain, pain with sex, discomfort with sitting, tailbone and low back pain, or even constipation.

The DIP Cycle

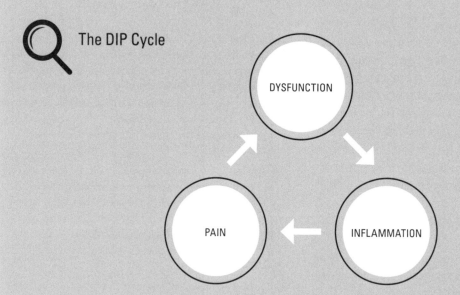

When I work with patients, I use the acronym "DIP" to remind them about the vicious cycle that we have to interrupt to restore normal function and relieve IC symptoms.

Dysfunction refers to any impairment or issue with normal operations of the body. For example, a catch in the knee causes a limp—the whole system from foot to hip is now dysfunctional. This happens within the pelvic floor as well. Your body has a mechanism by which it warns you when things are breaking down and not working right. It notifies your brain through pain. If something is damaged by the dysfunction, the body responds with inflammation.

Inflammation is the body's first responder. It is designed to clear out the problem areas and jumpstart the healing process. This works great for acute injuries, such as a sprained ankle. But when the damage is long-term and

continuous, more inflammation reaches the region than can be removed. The presence of inflammation tightens the muscles, causing further dysfunction and pain, which signals the brain to send even more inflammation.

Pain is a signal that notifies the brain of a potentially damaging situation. It can be external, like touching a hot stove, or something going wrong internally. When working properly, the pain system is sending you messages that encourage you to do the smart thing. Stop touching the hot stove, stop walking on the injured knee, and let the body heal. It is responsible for notifying the brain to send in the inflammatory response. Pain can also cause dysfunction, as the body seeks to compensate for the damaged or painful area.

What Causes Pelvic Floor Dysfunction?

The increased strain on your bladder and urethra from interstitial cystitis can cause pelvic floor dysfunction, but your pelvic floor dysfunction may have many other causes, as well. Studies focusing on elite athletes show that nearly half experience urinary incontinence stemming from pelvic floor dysfunction, indicating that severe physical strain can be a factor. Because all the pelvic floor muscles are connected to your pelvis, your posture can affect the ways in which those muscles stretch and tighten. Trauma to the region, such as falling on your tailbone, can also upset the delicate balance of the pelvic floor. Childbirth is another major cause of trauma to the area, and pelvic surgeries, such as C-sections, hysterectomies, or prostatectomies, frequently result in pelvic floor problems. Even something as simple as weakness in your core muscles can result in pelvic floor dysfunction. All these factors, among others, can contribute to pelvic floor muscle spasm and to your symptoms.

It is encouraging, too, that helping your pelvic floor can result in major, even unexpected, benefits. Lingering back pain or constipation problems may begin to fade. Or, you might feel stronger and have more energy. Your balance may improve. These pelvic floor issues often lurk just beneath the surface—they're not quite bad enough for us to realize they're there until we start to improve them and, in turn, notice improvements in other areas.

Patient's Story: IC Underlying Pelvic Floor Dysfunction

Jessica had come into my clinic with complaints of pain with sex that was interfering with her relationship with her fiancé. Her pelvic floor was extremely tight (hypertonic), so we worked to release the tension in the muscles surrounding the pelvis and, eventually, internally, as well. She developed a self-care routine, reducing her visits to once or twice a month. Best of all, she was able to resume intercourse with her partner in time for their honeymoon.

Jessica had also reported some urinary symptoms during treatment, but they weren't a primary focus. However, shortly after we resolved her sexual pain, she experienced a flare in these symptoms when she travelled: She was forced to sit a great deal and wasn't eating as well as usual. After an IC diagnosis she returned to physical therapy, where we addressed her new symptoms.

Did Jessica just suddenly develop IC? I don't believe so. Some researchers believe that IC actually underlies many other pelvic pain conditions. Patients with other pelvic floor problems are significantly more likely to be diagnosed with IC. In Jessica's case, her sexual pain was likely the first symptom of her IC.

What Helps the Pelvic Floor?

Fortunately, we can do quite a bit to help the pelvic floor function normally again. Pelvic floor dysfunction causes tightness in the muscles surrounding the region—in the abdomen, lower back, and thighs. By working to release the tension in these areas, the pelvic floor can be improved substantially. It's also important to strengthen weak core muscles to prevent problems from recurring. Techniques for helping the pelvic floor are found in chapters 9 and 10. Here are some ways to promote pelvic floor health.

- **Trigger point release** is a technique that works out the tight areas of a muscle to restore it to its normal length and function. These trigger points can be external—in the muscles connecting to the pelvis in the thighs, back, and abdomen—or internal. Internal trigger points can also be treated successfully at home with a simple program that releases the stress in the muscles.

- **Pelvic floor physical therapy** is a growing specialty in the field that can benefit interstitial cystitis patients and those with pelvic floor dysfunction. A properly trained therapist can address both the internal and external trigger points, release tension from the surrounding regions, and help your pelvic floor function normally again.

- **Changes in your daily routine and posture** can also have major effects on the pelvic floor. IC patients typically suffer when they sit for too long, which puts additional strain on the nerves of the pelvic floor. Many patients with pelvic floor dysfunction modify their workstations or find other ways to optimize their posture to reduce strain on the pelvic region.

Whether you do them alone or with a physical therapist, these techniques are the only treatment for interstitial cystitis proven to provide lasting and sustainable benefits for the majority of patients. By addressing the pelvic floor directly, you can reduce the symptoms of pain, urinary frequency, and other problems associated with IC. You may even find yourself eliminating symptoms you didn't even know were related to your condition.

Takeaways

- **All roads lead to the pelvic floor.** The pelvis lies at the intersection of the legs, back, and abdomen. The largest and most powerful muscles in the body connect there, but a tiny group of pelvic floor muscles also has a vital role to play. The pelvic floor supports the bladder and controls urination, and interstitial cystitis is a complex entanglement of pelvic floor and bladder dysfunction. Many "bladder" symptoms actually emanate from the pelvic floor.

- **Complete recovery from IC is impossible without addressing the pelvic floor.** In nearly all interstitial cystitis patients, a portion of symptoms stems from the bladder, while others arise from problems within the pelvic floor. Tension in the muscles surrounding the bladder can create or exacerbate IC symptoms, and a major part of your IC journey will involve resolving pelvic floor dysfunction and employing habits that promote a healthy pelvic floor.

SECTION II

Treatments and Therapies

6

TREATMENT OF IC:
An Overview

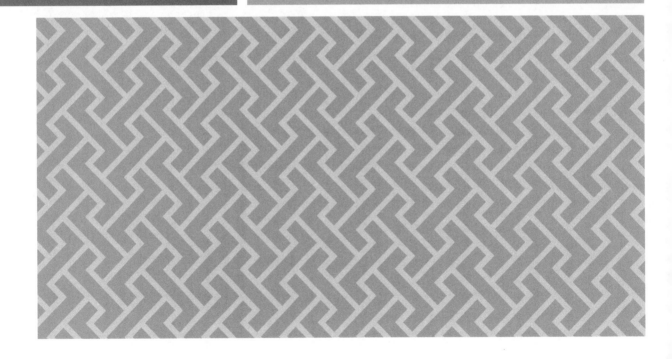

Successful healing with interstitial cystitis requires a balanced, holistic approach, and a combination of therapies is always required when dealing with such a complex condition. While there are many available treatments for IC, there's no single, universal cure that works for everyone. So part of your IC journey will be finding out what works for you, and what doesn't. And, the good news is, that there's certainly something that will work for you! This chapter gives you a brief rundown of treatment methods for interstitial cystitis, plus some guidelines for reviewing clinical studies when you're doing research on the condition.

First, a word to the wise: When you try any particular treatment, make sure you give it a chance to work. Some treatments will let you know almost immediately whether or not they'll be beneficial, while others can take weeks, or even months, to be fully effective. Keep this in mind, and evaluate whether you've given the treatment enough time: If it doesn't work for you, move on to the next option.

Many patients give up on promising therapies too early, before they could be expected to work. Some patients visit an inexperienced physical therapist for two sessions, see no immediate benefit, and, mistakenly, conclude that physical therapy won't be helpful for them. On the other hand, if you've been taking an oral medication for several months and have seen no improvements, it may be time to try something new. Certain treatments, such as acupuncture or nerve stimulation, recommend at least ten visits for full effect, while bladder instillations should give almost instantaneous relief if they are effective.

Interstitial cystitis is a complex condition that entangles the bladder, pelvic floor, and nervous system. The patients who have the most success in treating IC are the ones willing to try different types of therapy, and who persevere in trying alternatives until they discover their best treatment options.

Patient Story:
Finding a Treatment Plan

Robert came to my clinic after struggling with an IC diagnosis and pain for nearly a year. His doctor had originally only prescribed Elmiron, a common medication for treating IC. Unfortunately, it takes nearly six months to determine whether the drug will be beneficial, and it didn't help Robert. We helped him find a urologist who specializes in IC, as well as a pain-management doctor for his chronic pain.

A diligent patient, Robert started with a trial-and-error approach to the different medications his doctors recommended. He compared the benefits of different drugs with their side effects, and within a few months he had a treatment regimen that was working for him.

Robert was on three oral medications—an antidepressant to dampen his nervous system, a muscle relaxant to help with his pelvic floor muscle spasms, and an over-the-counter antihistamine to reduce inflammation. His pain-management doctor also prescribed an opioid medication to use as needed during flares. Robert realized that bladder instillations weren't helping very much, so he began trying neurostimulation. He came to physical therapy twice a week to clear the trigger points that were a major cause of his pain, and did a stretching routine at home. After learning about the effect diet can have on IC, he started the elimination diet, and realized alcohol and caffeine were his primary triggers.

This is the kind of holistic treatment approach that yields the best results; it requires perseverance and a trial-and-error approach, but it certainly makes healing possible.

Oral Medications

No single pharmaceutical remedy has emerged as a consensus treatment for interstitial cystitis. More than 180 different drugs have been proposed and tested for use in the condition, and only a single oral medication has been approved by the FDA for IC. Many drugs intended for other conditions are used off label (used in a different way from that described on the FDA-approved drug label), including medications for depression, antihistamines, and immunosuppressants.

Each drug can benefit a subset of patients, but there's no way to know which one will work for you in advance. You'll have to adopt that trial-and-error approach we keep mentioning. And, when it comes to drugs, side effects are also an important consideration. Your treatment will need to strike a balance between reaping the benefits of the drugs and minimizing their undesirable effects. Many of these medications focus on decreasing pain, which can help break the negative cycle of the condition and reverse nervous system upregulation.

Bladder and Medical Treatments

Bladder instillations deliver medication directly to the bladder through a catheter. In this way the drugs can reach the bladder lining and work to reduce bladder symptoms at the source. If there are wounds within the bladder lining, they can be cauterized during a medical procedure, which has been shown to bring relief to the small subset of patients with Hunner's lesions. Other medical procedures, such as nerve stimulation and numbing injections into the bladder, are beneficial for many IC patients.

Pelvic Floor Physical Therapy

The only treatment for interstitial cystitis shown to be consistently effective for a majority of IC patients is pelvic floor physical therapy. Manual physical therapy is the sole treatment given an "A" evidence grade by the American Urological Association, and is among the first medical interventions recommended for patients. Pelvic floor dysfunction is extremely common with IC, exacerbating existing symptoms and causing new ones. By addressing the tightness in the pelvic muscles, pelvic floor physical therapy alleviates symptoms and breaks the dysfunction–inflammation–pain cycle.

Self-Care Regimen

A self-care regimen of stretching and strengthening builds on pelvic floor physical therapy and works to eliminate symptoms caused by tight and knotted pelvic muscles. Deep breathing relaxes the pelvic floor and calms the nervous system. Stretching the muscles that connect to the pelvis reduces stress throughout the region. These self-care techniques can be done at home and benefit many patients.

Elimination Diet

The vast majority of IC patients have at least some sensitivity to certain foods and drinks that can trigger symptoms. The number of usual culprits is relatively small, and eliminating these foods from the diet can reduce the symptoms they trigger. There is no prescribed diet or specific set of rules for interstitial cystitis, but you can focus on eliminating foods that cause flares and, instead, on enjoying a varied, healthy diet.

Complementary and Alternative Medicine

This is a broad term for nontraditional therapies, and includes such treatments as acupuncture, nutritional supplements, vitamins, and other remedies. While many of these alternative approaches have not been rigorously evaluated, there are some that have been shown to have similar benefits to prescription medication, with fewer side effects. The border between these alternative treatments and the standard of care for the condition is fluid: It's constantly changing as new research is conducted. Some treatments considered "alternative" just a few years ago are now universally accepted.

Developing positive mental health and reducing stress can be invaluable when dealing with a chronic condition. Meditation, for instance, can actually rewire the brain to reduce pain levels. Cognitive behavioral therapy (CBT) trains patients to create better mental and physical habits to help them respond to IC. Psychotherapy, or even a supportive spouse or friend, can also play a significant role in your recovery. Taking care of your mental and emotional health can help improve your symptoms and overall well-being, which, in turn, makes you happier and more energetic. In this way, you can create a positive feedback loop that promotes healing by addressing both mental and physical health.

AMERICAN UROLOGICAL ASSOCIATION IC GUIDELINES

First line treatments	Education	Self-care and behavioral modification	Stress management
Second line treatments	Pelvic floor physical therapy	Oral medications (amitriptyline, cimetidine, hydroxyzine, or PPS)	Intravesical treatments (DMSO, heparin, lidocaine)
Third line treatments	Hydrodistention of the bladder	Fulguration of Hunner's lesions	
Fourth line treatments	Intradetrusor BOTOX	Neurostimulation	
Fifth line treatments	Cyclosporine A		
Sixth line treatments	Major surgery		
Not to be offered	Long-term antibiotics	Intravesical Bacillus Calmette-Guérin (BCG)	High-pressure, long-duration hydrodistention

The American Urological Association first published guidelines for the treatment of interstitial cystitis in 2011. It recommends a series of treatments to be followed as "lines" in order from conservative to aggressive. It's best to try the least-invasive treatments first and take more serious measures only if symptoms and pain cannot be controlled successfully. The guidelines also indicate outdated treatments that should not be tried by patients under any circumstances. If your doctor recommends one of these treatments, seek a second opinion before proceeding.

Reading and Understanding a Clinical Trial

You'll do a lot of your own research as part of your IC journey. You may come across clinical trials of new procedures, drugs, or treatments, and it can be difficult to understand the most important parts of these articles. Following is a summary of the most important aspects of a good study to help you determine whether a treatment or medication is likely to work for you.

Controlled Study

A control group in a study consists of patients who do not receive the treatment being evaluated: They'll often receive a placebo pill or sham treatment instead. Having a control group is one of the most important aspects of a good study, since it's used to rule out the placebo effect (see the following).

▪ Placebo Effect

The mind can have a powerful effect on the body—when you expect to get better, sometimes you actually do, regardless of what's physically happening. To that end, a placebo is a fake treatment—historically a sugar pill—that the patient believes is important medication. If research doesn't account for this effect, you can't be sure whether it's the treatment that's helping, or just the *belief* that the medication will help.

Placebos are designed to mimic the actual treatment so patients don't know whether they have received the real treatment or the fake one. This is called a blinded study. In the best studies, even the researchers don't know which patients receive the real drug or the placebo: These are called double-blinded studies.

 The Placebo Effect in Action

In one of the most famous examples of the placebo effect, researchers threw a keg party at a college that had the typical results: students (over twenty-one) stumbling around and talking with slurred speech and plenty of hangovers the next day. The only catch? The beer in the kegs was actually nonalcoholic. The students expected to be drunk, and their bodies fulfilled their expectations.

▪ Randomized

A controlled clinical trial should randomly assign patients to either the control or experimental group. Randomizing the process prevents bias from creeping in, when researchers might inadvertently select "better" patients to receive the treatment instead of the placebo.

What Is Statistical Significance?

When reading about scientific studies or articles, you'll run into the term "statistically significant." Simply put, if the results are statistically significant, the researchers are at least 95 percent sure they didn't happen by chance. The easiest example of this is flipping a coin. If you flip a coin once and publish your results, you'd report that the coin lands on heads or tails 100 percent of the time. However, because of the small sample size, your results were probably due to chance, and so they wouldn't be statistically significant. If, however, you flipped a coin one hundred times and it landed on heads each time, those results would be significant because you've seen it happen frequently enough to be sure it's not random chance.

If a study doesn't give statistically significant results should it be discounted? Not necessarily. Often—especially in studies involving IC, for which researchers have trouble finding enough patients—there is only a small number of patients in each study. In these cases, even a very beneficial drug or treatment may not yield statistically significant results.

Bias in Studies

As much as we try to prevent it, bias can creep into studies. After all, almost all studies are funded by a drug manufacturer or device manufacturer, and the study may have (unconsciously or consciously) been designed to favor the product in question. Plus, researchers don't usually write up (and journals don't publish) studies that demonstrate no benefit of a treatment. In fact, unsuccessful clinical trials are often simply shut down as soon as it becomes apparent they aren't working. That means that more than half of all clinical trials are never published.

For example, in one study of the published literature, researchers found that 94 percent of published clinical trials with antidepressants showed positive results. However, when they examined all the studies, including unpublished ones, that number dropped to only 51 percent. All negative trials were invisible to the doctors, researchers, and patients relying on the antidepressants.

Also, the authors of research papers are required to disclose their financial interest, so you should note the funding source. Again, this doesn't mean that a study by a manufacturer should be discounted, but it does mean you should approach the information with some skepticism and be sure it's a well-controlled, randomized, and blinded study before relying on its results.

Takeaways

- **A holistic approach to treatment gives the best results.** No single treatment or medication will eliminate your symptoms or cure interstitial cystitis on its own. By combining different treatments, you can improve the various aspects of the condition and get significant, sustained healing.

- **Trial and error is necessary.** It's impossible to know what will work best for you in advance, so the only way to find out is to try different treatment options. This will result in some wrong turns, but they are an important part of your journey. Make sure to give treatments sufficient time to work—but don't spend unnecessary time following a false trail.

7

A BITTER PILL:

Why Medication Isn't the Only Answer

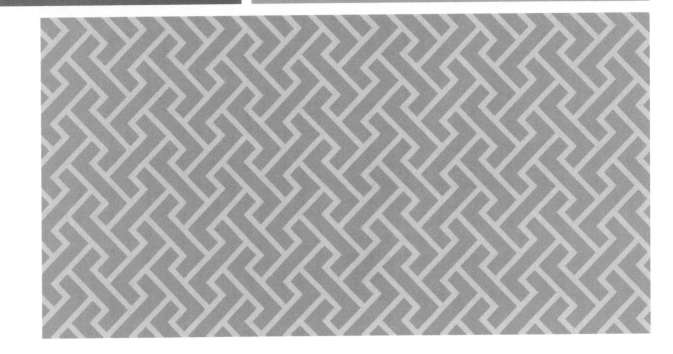

mericans consume a staggering amount of medication each year. Even though we comprise less than 5 percent of the world's population, we consume 75 percent of the world's prescription drugs, 80 percent of its pain medication, and 99 percent of its Vicodin (or generic equivalent). With three out of four visits to the doctor ending with a prescription for drugs, it's not surprising that half of Americans are on at least one medication. A recent study found that nearly 20 percent of the population is currently taking more than five medications at once. And that's only counting prescription drugs! Those statistics don't include all over-the-counter (OTC) options available, such as aspirin, ibuprofen, naproxen, and Tylenol, which 20 to 30 percent of Americans regularly use, taking an average of more than one hundred doses each year.

Despite all the medication, Americans live in far more pain than their counterparts elsewhere in the developed world. One hundred million Americans—more than one in three—struggle with chronic pain, a rate nearly double that of Europe. If chronic pain could be cured with painkillers and prescriptions, we would have eradicated it long ago.

By the time you've been diagnosed with IC, it's likely your body is entangled in a complex feedback loop that includes the bladder, inflammatory response, nervous system, pelvic floor muscles, and the psychological impact of chronic pain. No single medication is able to address all the different facets of the condition and resolve the underlying issue. So, as you'll learn in this chapter, we need to change our thinking when it comes to chronic pain—specifically when that pain accompanies interstitial cystitis.

 Off-Label Medications

Almost all oral medications typically used for interstitial cystitis were originally designed, tested, and approved for other conditions. It is completely legal and commonplace for a doctor to prescribe these drugs for off-label uses, but they have not been evaluated by the Food and Drug Administration (FDA) for their effectiveness in treating IC. These drugs have often been shown to reduce pain in other chronic conditions or have another effect that could help in treating IC symptoms.

Oral medication can be an important component of IC treatment. Medications can reduce pain and help reset that vicious cycle of pain, urinary symptoms, and inflammation that makes IC so hard to treat. Successful pain treatment can help reverse nervous system upregulation—and, when you're in less pain, you're better able to focus on other treatments that can address some of the underlying issues. Breaking the pain cycle is especially important early on in your interstitial cystitis journey, or when dealing with a symptom flare. At both times it's important to do everything you can, including taking oral medications, to reduce pain and inflammation.

Many of these medications can have significant adverse effects. Sometimes these side effects can actually be helpful—for example, antihistamines are famous for making you drowsy, which can be desirable around bedtime—but other times they can be nearly as bad as the symptoms themselves. In some cases, the side effects are specifically detrimental for IC patients. For instance, some antidepressants used for pain management can cause urinary retention, which might not be a major problem for a patient with a healthy bladder—but it can be highly problematic for someone with interstitial cystitis. Constipation is another common side effect of many medications that can exacerbate a problem many people with IC already face. There is no good way to know which medications you'll be most responsive to, or which will cause the greatest side effects, so determining which combination of oral medications works best for you is done by trial and error.

The American Urological Association's guidelines grade the oral medications that have been tested for the treatment of IC. Each medication is ranked in a line of treatment, which indicates the order in which the AUA recommends trying it. They are also given evidence grades, based on the quality and quantity of scientific research that supports their efficacy for treating interstitial cystitis. You may not see a medication your doctor has recommended on this list. Many of the commonly prescribed oral medications have not been specifically tested in IC patients, and so have not been evaluated by the AUA. This doesn't mean they can't be effective in reducing pain or inflammation—they often have been tested for use with other chronic pain conditions—only that they haven't been evaluated directly against interstitial cystitis. Always consult with your doctor or specialist to determine your course of treatment.

AMERICAN UROLOGICAL ASSOCIATION'S ORAL MEDICATION GRADES FOR IC

Name	Type	Trade names	AUA line of treatment	AUA evidence grade
Amitriptyline	Antidepressant	Elavil	II	B
Cimetidine	Antihistamine	Tagamet	II	B
Hydroxyzine	Antihistamine/ anti-anxiety	Vistaril, Atarax	II	C
Pentosan Polysulfate	Similar to anticoagulants	Elmiron, PPS	II	B
Cyclosporine A	Immunosuppressant	CyA	V	C

Over-the-Counter Pain Medications

Most people turn first to over-the-counter drugs for pain relief. Many fall into the NSAID (nonsteroidal anti-inflammatory drugs) category, which includes aspirin, ibuprofen, and naproxen. Here's how they work: When your body perceives an injury at a specific site, it responds by swelling. This inflammation amplifies the pain signals from the region, making sure your brain pays attention to the problem. These drugs go right to the source, preventing this swelling from occurring at the painful site. The other common OTC painkiller is acetaminophen (Tylenol), which has less of an effect on local pain and a more general effect on the nervous system.

Although these drugs are widely used and available, they are not without risks and side effects. For example, gastrointestinal irritation is common with long-term NSAID use, and can be particularly relevant to IC patients with Irritable Bowel Syndrome. And some OTC painkillers are not recommended for patients with kidney problems. Remember to mention your OTC drugs to your doctor to make sure they won't increase your risk of side effects or negatively interact with any prescription medication you take.

Oral Urinary Tract Analgesics

Certain oral medications have a pain-killing effect directly on the lining of the urethra. Designed to reduce pain from UTIs or invasive bladder procedures, such as cystoscopies, they deliver an analgesic into the urine, which then coats the urethra during urination. These medications include phenazopyridine (Azo, Pyridium) and Uribel. Both prescription and OTC versions are available.

These medications are most helpful for patients who experience burning in the urethra, and urgency and difficulty in urinating. However, they are not long-term solutions, because it's hard for the kidneys to process these drugs. They are most beneficial during pain flares or before undergoing a cystoscopy or bladder instillation. In studies on UTI patients, the medication's peak benefit was seen approximately five hours after it was taken, so you can see a rapid effect.

The most visible side effect of these drugs is that they turn your urine a different color: a burnt orange for phenazopyridine (Pyridium) or blue for Uribel. Be careful: These colors will stain fabrics or anything else they touch. Other side effects include headache, dizziness, and an upset stomach. Also, it's best to take this medication on a full stomach.

 ## Patient Story: Medications

Emily had been diagnosed with fibromyalgia and IC. She had been prescribed an antidepressant that dampened her nervous system and reduced her fibromyalgia pain. She continued with physical therapy for her IC, and, after a few months, was feeling much better. But she didn't like the side effects of her medications, and wanted to reduce the number of pharmaceuticals she was taking as soon as possible.

With her fibromyalgia under control and her IC improving rapidly, she decided to go off the antidepressant. Her symptoms immediately flared, and it took her almost four months—and a return to the medication—to get back to where she had been. Many medications used to treat fibromyalgia and IC are prescribed for both conditions. So don't assume the medication you're taking "for your [fill in the blank]" isn't having a positive effect on your IC and overall health. Managing pain in one area can be therapeutic for pain in another.

Antidepressant Medication

Antidepressants are used to treat IC, typically at lower doses than prescribed for clinical depression because they can dampen the nervous system. One of the biggest challenges with IC is the upregulation of the nervous system, in which normal sensations are interpreted by the brain as pain. An antidepressant may calm the nerves and help restore normal responses to pain. It may take several weeks or longer to notice a difference. They can be an important part of your treatment plan, particularly early in your IC journey, by helping disrupt the cycle of pain and symptoms—but even when they work well, they aren't enough to address all the symptoms of IC. Antidepressants are best used in combination with other medication and treatments that work to resolve the underlying causes of IC pain.

Antidepressants are an obvious option if you struggle with depression along with interstitial cystitis, as chronic medical conditions are associated with a higher risk of depression and anxiety. If you do experience signs of clinical depression, such medications may help both your emotional and physical health.

Amitriptyline is one of the most common antidepressants used off-label for treating IC. Two controlled and randomized clinical studies have been conducted with the drug for IC. A 2010 study funded by the National Institutes of Health showed that 55 percent of people who took the drug moderately or markedly improved, which was only 10 percent higher than the results of the placebo group; the difference between the two wasn't statistically significant. The drug also has a high rate of adverse effects that can affect as many as 80 percent of patients as reported in several studies—though most were relatively mild, and included fatigue, gastrointestinal issues, and dizziness. Patients who take it solely for depression tolerate these side effects for long periods of use.

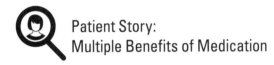

Patient Story: Multiple Benefits of Medication

Esther, a patient with interstitial cystitis, was so upset by her diagnosis that she couldn't talk about her symptoms in physical therapy without crying. When I first met her, she was in constant 6-out-of-10 pain. She had trouble sleeping, and constant exhaustion played a role in exacerbating her symptoms.

Her doctor prescribed Cymbalta, a common antidepressant, which helped with emotional coping and her physical pain. As the medication reduced the upregulation of her nervous system and stabilized her moods, her pain began to decrease.

The medication didn't eliminate her pain or symptoms completely. Esther still needed several months of physical therapy and a self-care program, among other treatments, to control her condition. But the oral medication lowered her pain to a manageable level, allowing her to concentrate on her physical therapy and address the underlying causes of her symptoms.

The authors noted that if patients are able to tolerate the side effects, doses higher than 50 mg per day were more effective and had a statistically significant improvement over the placebo. The American Urologic Association lists amitriptyline as a second-line medication, and gave it a "B" for evidence of safety and efficacy.

Amitriptyline (Elavil) is the only antidepressant specifically studied for use in the treatment of IC and named in the AUA guidelines, but it is part of a class of drugs called tricyclic antidepressants (TCAs). Others in this category include imipramine (Tofranil), clomipramine (Anafranil), sinequan (Doxepin), nortriptyline (Pamelor), and desipramine (Norpramin). These are all thought to work in the same way that amitriptyline does, so consult your doctor to determine which may be the right option for you.

Another class of antidepressants that is commonly prescribed for chronic pain is called serotonin-norepinephrine reuptake inhibitors (SNRIs). The two drugs from this category that are often prescribed for chronic pain are duloxetine (Cymbalta) and milnacipran (Savella). Both drugs have been approved in the treatment of fibromyalgia, which shares important characteristics, and often overlaps, with interstitial cystitis. This class of drugs is more targeted than TCAs, and some patients report they experience less drowsiness with these types of antidepressants. Duloxetine has been used to reduce urinary stress incontinence, which can have a negative effect on some IC patients because it may cause urinary retention.

A similar class of drugs is gabapentinoids. These drugs are not prescribed for depression, but, typically, are used to reduce nerve pain. Of these, pregabalin (Lyrica) and gabapentin (Neurontin) are the most commonly prescribed. They're approved for neuropathic pain or fibromyalgia, and gabapentin has also been used to treat anxiety disorders. Drowsiness is a common side effect.

There are many considerations when selecting an antidepressant. All have significant side effects that vary from patient to patient, and it's important to choose the one with the most-tolerable side effects for you. As noted, only one antidepressant, amitriptyline, has been specifically tested in IC patients. However, many of these drugs have approvals for neuropathic pain conditions, chronic pain, or fibromyalgia and can be effective in reducing pain and reversing nervous system upregulation.

 Advocates for IC

The Interstitial Cystitis Association (ICA) was founded by medical student Vicki Ratner in 1984. Struggling with unexplained bladder pain and symptoms, she diagnosed herself with interstitial cystitis and set out on a mission to educate the medical community and the general population about the disease.

In 1987, the National Institutes of Health published the first formal definition of interstitial cystitis. The ICA has been instrumental in obtaining funding and support for research in the field.

Some of these drugs have been on the market for a long time and generic versions are available, which are substantially less expensive than brand-name drugs. When discussing options with your doctor, don't be afraid to mention your concerns about the cost of a medication. There's generally a generic version in each of these major antidepressant categories, and your doctor can direct you to them. (For more information on treating IC on a budget, see page 198.) Finding the right medication and dosage will require some trial and error, so don't be afraid to ask your doctor for a different option if the drug you've been prescribed isn't working for you.

Antihistamine Medication

Histamine is a central component of the inflammatory response, rushing the body's first responders to the site of an injury. In chronic conditions, inflammation is sent to the damaged area of the body faster than it can be cleared away, amassing in the area and causing additional problems. Lingering inflammation can trigger additional pain and dysfunction, which then causes the body to create even more inflammation.

Antihistamine medications are designed to break one point of that loop by reducing the inflammatory response. We often associate these medications with the treatment of allergies, but they have a similar effect when used in chronic pain conditions, such as interstitial cystitis. Antihistamines have a well-deserved reputation for side effects, particularly drowsiness. Many patients actually harness that side effect and take their medication before bed, allowing the sedation of the antihistamine to help them fall and stay asleep.

One of the few antihistamines formally evaluated for interstitial cystitis, cimetidine (Tagamet), also blocks the production of stomach acid. Typically prescribed for heartburn or peptic ulcers, researchers thought cimetidine might be able to restore the bladder lining (GAG layer). In a well-designed clinical trial published in 2001, the London-based authors found that three months of treatment with cimetidine reduced overall symptoms of IC by nearly 40 percent, demonstrating a significant benefit over the 3.5 percent improvement with the placebo. The number of nighttime bathroom visits decreased from an average of three times a night to once. Suprapubic pain was also significantly lowered in patients that received the drug. Interestingly, the authors showed that it had no effect on the bladder lining—their initial hypothesis—but it helped patients anyway. It also showed relatively low levels of adverse effects, which may make it an interesting option for patients who experience unwanted side effects with other medications. The AUA considers cimetidine a second-line option in the treatment of IC, and rates the evidence for effectiveness as a "B."

Several other antihistamines in the same class as cimetidine may also be options for IC patients, such as ranitidine (Zantac), which is available as an over-the-counter medication. Famotidine (Pepcid), another histamine inhibitor, is available as both a prescription medication or as an OTC. All three drugs work to affect the same histamine receptor, and all may be options for IC treatment.

Then there's hydroxyzine, an antihistamine that's often prescribed as an anti-anxiety medication or used to treat allergic conditions. Unlike cimetidine, it does not have a significant effect on the production of stomach acid. In a single clinical trial with a small number of patients conducted over six months, 31 percent of patients taking hydroxyzine showed clinically significant improvement, as compared to 20 percent for the placebo—an effect that wasn't statistically significant. However, additional research in uncontrolled studies showed that hydroxyzine was much more effective in IC patients who had systemic allergies, suggesting that the drug may be more effective in a small subset of IC patients. More than 80 percent of patients reported side effects from it, including drowsiness, dizziness, dry mouth, and constipation. The AUA Guidelines list hydroxyzine as a second-line treatment, and give the drug a "C" for evidence of efficacy.

While these are the only two antihistamines formally evaluated in clinical trials and by the American Urological Association guidelines, there are many different antihistamines that work in similar ways. Over-the-counter medications are generally not as strong, but also are less prone to side effects and are less expensive than prescription drugs.

Pentosan Polysulfate (PPS, Elmiron)

The only FDA-approved oral medication for the treatment of IC, PPS received FDA approval in 1996. It is, by far, the most-studied oral medication for interstitial cystitis: Seven controlled clinical trials have evaluated the drug in more than 500 patients.

However, the results of these studies have been contradictory, and the drug seems to benefit only a small subset of patients. In the studies in which PPS was shown to be significantly better than the placebo, it was still only showing a clinical benefit for 28 to 32 percent of patients (as compared to 13 to 16 percent for a placebo). In a study comparing PPS against another drug, Cyclosporine A (CyA), PPS showed improvement in just 19 percent of patients, while CyA was effective for 75 percent. Several studies showed no significant benefit over a placebo.

One other interesting aspect of PPS is that many patients may be taking more of the medication than necessary, which can increase the potential for side effects. One published dose-dependent study showed no significant increase in efficacy when the drug was increased from 300 to 900 mg. Another study, an unpublished clinical trial that was abandoned because the drug wasn't showing a benefit (as reported by the AUA), showed there was no major difference in efficacy between a daily dose of 100 mg and 300 mg of the drug.

A significant drawback of PPS is that it can take a long time to know whether you respond positively to the drug. In one study, fewer than 20 percent of patients were considered to be responders after four weeks, but after the full trial of nearly eight months, that number had more than doubled. Most patients who take the drug will not respond within the first few months, and a longer course is required to see improvement. So, doctors usually ask their patients to take the drug for four to six months to determine whether it helps. Some patients may find this difficult, since they might experience side effects—including hair loss, nausea, diarrhea, and headaches—before the treatment becomes effective, and even then it won't be effective in more than half of those who take it. However, for those who do see a benefit, PPS can be an important medication in successful IC treatment.

Cyclosporine A (CyA)

Cyclosporine A is a high-risk treatment for interstitial cystitis. Typically used as an immunosuppressant during organ transplants, CyA has also been prescribed to treat rheumatoid arthritis and ulcerative colitis. In clinical studies, it demonstrated some of the most dramatic benefits of any of the oral medications studied, but it also has a high rate of adverse events—many of them severe.

When Finnish researchers conducted a comparison study against PPS, Cyclosporine A was found to help 75 percent of patients, while the more commonly prescribed PPS was only beneficial in 19 percent of patients. However, 94 percent of the patients treated with CyA reported adverse events, as compared with the (still-high) rate of 56 percent for PPS. In other studies, CyA showed improvement in nearly 60 percent of patients, but, again, this was accompanied by high rates of serious adverse events, such as high blood pressure, facial and body hair growth, ulcers in the mouth, headaches, nausea, and vomiting. CyA is also known to be very hard on the kidneys and liver. Because of the potential for adverse events, the AUA lists Cyclosporine A as a fifth-line treatment, only to be tried—with caution—after a patient hasn't experienced substantial success with other treatments and remedies.

Muscle Relaxants

One of the major challenges of interstitial cystitis is tight muscles in the pelvic floor that can create or amplify symptoms. Muscle relaxants are designed to reduce the spasm of these tight muscles. These drugs, including baclofen, diazepam, tizanidine, and dantrolene, actually work on the nerves and not the muscles. They affect the brain, brain stem, and spinal cord: By making it more difficult for your nerves to send signals to your muscles, they can ease the tension in those muscles.

An important 2013 study examined whether the muscle relaxant diazepam (Valium) was able to help an extremely tight (hypertonic) pelvic floor. No benefit was seen when patients were given suppositories for four weeks in the blinded, controlled study. However, when combined with pelvic floor physical therapy, 96 percent (25 of 26) patients saw improvement in their pelvic floor pain and symptoms. This data indicates that muscle relaxants by themselves may not be effective in helping the pelvic floor, but can *enhance* the benefits of physical therapy or self-care.

Although no clinical trials have been published to evaluate muscle relaxants specifically for interstitial cystitis, many patients report relief with these medications. They can be particularly beneficial if a tight pelvic floor or surrounding muscles in the legs are a primary cause of symptoms. Muscle relaxants may allow those muscles to be stretched and relaxed more easily, which can ease pain in the bladder and pelvic floor.

Muscle relaxants are often prescribed in suppository form. However, their entire effect is on the central nervous system—the brain and spinal cord. Studies have shown that the same amount enters the bloodstream whether you take the medication orally or in a rectal or vaginal suppository.

Opioid Painkillers

Opioids are a powerful class of painkillers typically prescribed only for patients with high pain levels that can't be controlled with other methods. Unlike antihistamines or other anti-inflammatory medications that work right at the source of pain, or antidepressants that can help reset the upregulated nervous system, opioids have no intrinsic benefit for interstitial cystitis. They simply mask the pain associated with the condition.

However, if you are in substantial pain from IC, opioids can be an important tool if you cannot perform your daily activities. Generally, a long-lasting opioid will be prescribed for daily use, along with a fast-acting supplemental medication for breakthrough pain. Many patients then transition to using a fast-acting opioid during major symptom flares, as needed.

There are substantial side effects to opioid medication, including the risk of dependency. If your pain is bad enough to require these painkillers, consider working with a pain-management specialist who is accustomed to opioid prescriptions and can gradually and safely increase your dosage to an effective amount. In addition to nausea and drowsiness, opioids are also notorious for causing constipation, which can be an aggravating aspect of interstitial cystitis. Though opioids should only be used as a treatment of last resort and are not a permanent solution, they can be an important tool for patients whose pain prevents them from going about the activities of daily life, and help with breakthrough flares.

Medical Marijuana

Although it may be a hot-button political issue, nearly half of the states in the United States have legalized the use of medical marijuana. It is often used to treat chronic pain, and some researchers believe cannabis can be more effective than traditional pain medications, with fewer associated side effects. Although there haven't been clinical trials specifically conducted with interstitial cystitis, medical marijuana has shown a benefit in chronic pain in multiple studies. In one review of eighteen different controlled clinical trials, patients reported a significant improvement in pain in fifteen of the studies, as well as improvements in sleep quality. No serious adverse events were reported, but mild or moderate side effects such as dizziness, dry mouth, and drowsiness are often reported.

In a clinical trial that tested cannabis for treating fibromyalgia, patients noted a significant reduction in pain and anxiety. In one clinical trial with chronic pain resulting from multiple sclerosis, cannabis was shown to reduce pain by more than 40 percent and prevented half of sleep disturbances. Some studies have reported that higher levels of the active ingredient result in more effective pain reduction, but with a corresponding increase in side effects. If you have difficulty controlling pain with traditional medications, and medical marijuana is legal in your state, it may be an option for breaking the pain cycle.

Oral Antibiotics

Some doctors have prescribed oral antibiotics for patients with interstitial cystitis without any evidence of an infection. The underlying premise seems to be that there might be undetectable bacteria in the bladder or urethra causing the symptoms—a theory that seems to be based on the similarities between the symptoms of IC and urinary tract infections. But no evidence has ever been found to support it, and oral antibiotics should *never* be used to treat interstitial cystitis. They are one of the few treatments that the American Urological Association specifically discourages. Antibiotics should only be used if you have been diagnosed with a bacterial infection: They should never be prescribed "just in case."

Now, it is possible to have a true UTI in addition to interstitial cystitis, and IC patients may actually have a higher risk of infection. In that case, antibiotics are necessary to eliminate the bacteria. If you have persistent recurring UTIs, your doctor may prescribe an ongoing, low-dose antibiotic to prevent these infections. Sometimes it can be hard to tell whether you are having a bad flare or have a UTI. UTI test strips that you can purchase for home use can help you discern the difference. Antibiotics should be used solely to combat or prevent bacterial infection; not as a treatment for interstitial cystitis.

Medication Response Time

Which oral medication will be most helpful for you? There's no obvious or easy answer to that question. No oral medication is beneficial for the majority of patients, and oral medications will only be one part of your entire treatment plan.

Consider how long it takes a medication to be effective when deciding which drug or drugs to try first. For example, most antidepressants are beneficial within two to three weeks. After a short trial, you can be certain—one way or the other—about the pros and cons of the medication. Oral bladder analgesics work within a few hours, so you will know almost immediately whether they help during a flare.

That's one reason I don't often advise a patient to start solely with a medication such as Elmiron: It takes six months to know for sure whether it's working or not. Like other medications, it doesn't show a benefit for the majority of patients, so, if it doesn't work for you, that's six months of lost recovery time. Alternatively, you could have tried six different antihistamines or antidepressants in that timeframe to find what works best for you while minimizing side effects. Give yourself the best odds of success—try different medications and pay attention to the time it will take to evaluate whether they work for you.

COMMON ORAL MEDICATIONS FOR IC

Name	Medications	Time to evaluate	Common side effects	Results in IC
OTC pain medications	• aspirin • ibuprofen • naproxen • Tylenol	immediate	upset stomach, rare kidney damage with extended use	Not tested.
Oral bladder analgesics	• phenazopyridine (Azo, Pyridium) • Uribel	immediate	headache, dizziness, upset stomach	Not tested; shown to be effective in reducing urethral pain from urinary tract infections and bladder procedures (catheterizations, cystoscopies).
Tricyclic antidepressants	• Anafranil • Doxepin • Elavil • Norpramin • Pamelor • Tofranil	4 weeks	fatigue, upset stomach, dizziness, dry mouth, weight gain	Forty-six percent of patients reported "excellent" or "good" satisfaction with results of amitriptyline treatment for IC.
SNRI antidepressants	• Cymbalta • Savella	4 weeks	nausea, dry mouth, constipation, drowsiness, dizziness	Not tested in IC; approved for fibromyalgia.
H-2 antihistamines	• Pepcid • Tagamet • Zantac	4 weeks	drowsiness, dizziness, headache, constipation	Tagamet showed a 40 percent reduction in IC symptoms (4 percent for placebo).
H-1 antihistamines	• Allegra • Benadryl • Claritin • hydroxyzine (Vistaril, Atarax)	4 weeks	drowsiness, dizziness, dry mouth, constipation	Thirty-one percent of IC patients showed improvement (20 percent for placebo).
Pentosan polysulfate (PPS)	• Elmiron	6 months	hair loss, itching, skin rash, diarrhea, nausea, dizziness, headache, upset stomach	Two clinical trials showed benefit in 28 to 32 percent of patients (13 to 16 percent of placebo). Two other controlled trials showed no significant benefit over placebo.

This table shows common oral medications for IC and the approximate length of time you should give each medication before deciding whether it works. Several of these medications start with a low dose and gradually increase. You may also notice side effects before you see the benefit of the treatment. Remember, these are general guidelines; always consult your doctor.

Name	Medications	Time to evaluate	Common side effects	Results in IC
Muscle relaxants	• baclofen • dantrolene • diazepam • tizanidine	2 to 4 weeks	weakness, drowsiness, dizziness, nausea, constipation	not tested for IC; has shown benefits for pelvic floor dysfunction in 96 percent of patients when taken in conjunction with pelvic floor physical therapy
Immunosuppressant	Cyclosporine A (CyA)	3 months	high blood pressure, facial and body hair growth, gout, ulcers, kidney and liver damage	75 percent of patients responded favorably to treatment (19 percent of PPS patients)
Opioid pain medication	• hydrocodone • oxycodone	immediate	drowsiness, dizziness, nausea, constipation, dry mouth	not tested in IC
Medical marijuana		immediate	impact on mental state, including memory, coordination, judgment, and balance	not tested in IC

Takeaways

- **Oral medication is important, but no single pill is the answer.** Oral medication will almost certainly be a part of your holistic treatment plan for interstitial cystitis, but it won't be the sole answer.

- **No medication works in the majority of patients.** Even when a medication is effective for you, it probably won't eliminate all symptoms. Finding the medication and dosage that delivers the most benefit with the fewest side effects is a process of trial and error. Talk to your doctor about the choices available.

- **Oral medications are like your hiking boots.** They are supportive and protective, and it may take some experimentation before you find your perfect fit. Still, your boots alone won't get you to your destination—that depends on your energy, perseverance, and willpower.

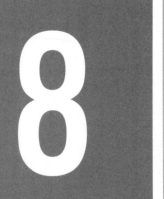

8

WITHIN THE BLADDER:

How Your Doctor Can Help

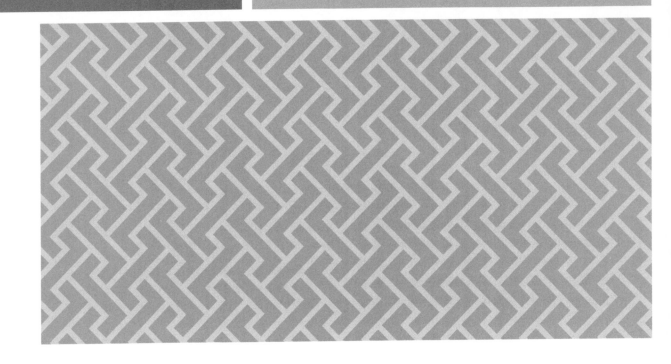

When we're in pain, we want to target the problem at its source. To that end, there are many medical procedures directly addressing the bladder that can be beneficial for interstitial cystitis, and they're often conducted by either urologists or urogynecologists. As with oral medications, most of these treatments are off-label and haven't been formally approved for IC, but they have shown benefits for patients in small clinical trials. And most treatments for the bladder are fast acting, so you'll know quickly whether they work for you or not.

The American Urological Association lists several methods in their guidelines for interstitial cystitis, and recommends that these procedures be tried in order, from the least invasive to the most intrusive. In the following chart, the AUA line column indicates the order in which treatments should be tried, while the AUA evidence grade column represents the quality and quantity of supporting evidence for the treatment.

AMERICAN UROLOGICAL ASSOCIATION GUIDELINES FOR IC BLADDER TREATMENTS

Name	Type	AUA line	AUA evidence grade
DMSO	Bladder instillation	II	C
Heparin	Bladder instillation	II	C
Lidocaine	Bladder instillation	II	B
Fulguration of Hunner's lesions	Bladder procedure	III	C
Hydrodistention (low pressure)	Bladder procedure	III	C
Intra-Bladder BOTOX (BTX-A)	Bladder injection	IV	C
InterStim	Neuromodulation	IV	C
Bladder removal surgery	Surgery	VI	C
BCG (bacillus Calmette-Guérin)	Bladder instillation	Not recommended	
Resiniferatoxin	Bladder instillation	Not recommended	

The AUA has published recommendations for patients to begin treatment with the most conservative options (Line II) and progress to other options if symptoms cannot be controlled.

"Bladder instillations are most effective when used to control pain and symptoms while you try other treatments to address the underlying condition."

Bladder Instillations

One of the earliest methods for treating interstitial cystitis involves applying medication directly to the bladder. The first FDA-approved IC treatment was a bladder instillation in 1978. To deliver the medication, a catheter is threaded up the urethra and into the bladder so that liquid medication can be directly infused. The benefit of these types of treatments is that they directly target the bladder. Oral medications, on the other hand, must pass through the stomach and intestines and into the bloodstream, and are diluted throughout the body before reaching the bladder.

Bladder instillations can be important tools for IC patients, mainly because they make it possible to apply pain-reducing medication directly to the inflamed bladder lining. Plus, instillations have been shown to reduce urinary urgency and frequency in some patients. And, unlike many oral medications for interstitial cystitis, bladder instillations typically have a rapid effect. Many patients notice symptom relief during the procedure itself, as the medication works directly on the bladder tissue.

This pain and symptom reduction can be useful if you're new to treatment, or if you struggle to control your pain levels. When pain is holding you back from other treatments—physical therapy, stretching, proper diet, moderate exercise—it needs to be reduced to a more manageable point. Bladder instillations can also counteract the extra pain that accompanies a bad flare.

However, current evidence suggests that bladder instillations offer few long-term healing effects. The benefits are present as long as the installations continue, but fade as soon as they are stopped. Therefore, bladder instillations are most effective when used to control pain and symptoms while you try other treatments to address the underlying condition.

The standard frequency of treatments is twice per week, since the effectiveness of many of the medications begins to wear off between three and seven days after treatment. So, as with all medications, let your body be your guide when it comes to bladder instillations. If the installation works well and you notice that symptoms are reduced for seven to ten days after the instillation, you can reduce your treatments to once per week. Once their condition is under control, some patients stop regular instillations but still use them during symptom flares.

Urethral Irritation with Bladder Instillations

Bladder instillations do have a downside—they're invasive. To perform them, a catheter must be inserted through the urethra, which can already be very irritated in IC patients. The physical insertion of this tube is the main source of side effects in bladder instillations, so that's a concern regardless of the type of medication applied. If you are already experiencing moderate or severe urethral pain, you may want to have it under control before using a catheter.

You can do several things to reduce the irritation caused by a catheter. Ask your doctor to use a pediatric-size tube, which may reduce painful contact with the urethra (although it will take slightly longer to complete the instillation). Also, ensure that the clinic you visit uses an anesthetic on the catheter itself. Some catheters come pretreated with a topical pain-killing medication. Alternatively, the nurse can coat it with lidocaine before the procedure to reduce pain. You can also take an oral bladder analgesic (see chapter 7) prior to the procedure to reduce pain. It will become apparent in the first few treatments if severe urethral irritation or other side effects will accompany your instillations.

After the medication is transferred into the bladder the catheter is removed and the patient is instructed to hold the liquid in the bladder for at least twenty minutes, or longer if possible. For some patients with strong urinary urgency, keeping the medication inside the bladder for this period of time is very difficult: Straining to hold in the medicine can be painful, or may cause the pelvic floor to clench, exacerbating symptoms. Sometimes the medication can help the bladder be less sensitive as it fills, which allows patients to hold the medication in for as long as two hours.

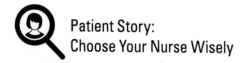

Patient Story: Choose Your Nurse Wisely

The nurse who inserts the catheter can have a huge effect on your experience with bladder instillations. Just as some nurses seem to have the knack for finding a vein on the first try when they take your blood, there's a level of skill and experience that's important when it comes to inserting the catheter. For example, I had one patient who was seeing good results with her instillations, which were being conducted by a nurse who had been performing the procedure for more than thirty years. But on the days when that nurse was off, my patient had severe post-procedure flares. After a few of these experiences, she specifically requested that the experienced nurse oversee all her bladder instillations, and made sure her appointments aligned with the nurse's schedule. Everyone's body is unique, and when the same person performs the instillation each time, he or she will become more adept at inserting the catheter.

Remember: Never be afraid to ask for something from your doctor or from any other medical practitioner. Your doctor sees hundreds of patients a year; you aren't going to offend her, and your health is much more important than the embarrassment of asking. In my patient's case, the clinic's staff was very glad that she spoke up, because otherwise she might have just stopped coming for treatment. They were happy to assign her to the more experienced nurse.

Which Bladder Instillation to Try?

There are several options for bladder instillations, but no consensus on a standard of care. These medications will typically be administered by a nurse in a urology or urogynecology clinic, but you can self-administer instillations if you are comfortable using the catheter. Some patients like doing it themselves because it gives them the freedom to use bladder instillations on their own schedules; others ask to self-administer for special circumstances, perhaps while on vacation. If you're interested in trying this, ask your doctor to teach you how to catheterize yourself and instill the medication, or to teach your significant other to do it instead.

Three different medications are recommended by the AUA as second-line treatments: DMSO, heparin, and lidocaine.

Each medication tends to help only a subset of patients, so many doctors have switched to "cocktails" of combined medications, which is a practical way to approach the problem. After all, everyone responds differently to IC treatments, so combining multiple medications maximizes your chances of responding favorably. Side effects generally stem from the procedure itself, not from the medication, so a cocktail approach offers more potential benefit without increasing the risk of adverse events. For instance, heparin and lidocaine are often used together, as they may have different mechanisms of action and help the bladder in two different ways. Some doctors prefer an even larger cocktail of drugs, believing it can only increase the chance of a successful treatment.

• DMSO

DMSO is the first and only drug that's been FDA-approved for bladder instillations in cases of interstitial cystitis. It received approval in 1978. In early clinical studies, it was shown to improve symptoms markedly in more than 50 percent of patients after only two instillations, as compared to improvement in 18 percent of those in the control group.

Another study compared DMSO to BCG (bacillus Calmette-Guérin) therapy, and, again, found improvement in approximately 50 percent of patients with DMSO as compared to none in the BCG group.

A third clinical trial found the rate of improvement with the drug was around 60 percent, with 7 percent of patients dropping out of the study due to adverse events.

Along with the irritation from the installation procedure, DMSO can also cause a burning sensation in the bladder. However, the primary side effect of DMSO therapy is that the drug is metabolized in the body into a compound that has an unpleasant odor. While it's safe to use, DMSO treatment results in an unappealing, sulfuric body odor on the skin and a garlicky aftertaste in the mouth that can persist for several days after treatment. Because of this malodorous effect, DMSO has fallen out of favor with many doctors and patients, although it still can be an effective option.

• **Heparin**

Heparin is another common medication in bladder installations that's used off-label for interstitial cystitis. Researchers hypothesize that it may temporarily reinforce the GAG layer of the bladder, which may be damaged in some IC patients. Like DMSO, heparin is listed by the AUA as a second-line treatment option with an evidence level of "C."

Uncontrolled studies have demonstrated clinical benefits of heparin therapy in a little over 50 percent of patients. One misconception some clinicians hold is that heparin may take a long time to be truly effective, but the fact is, like all instillation treatments, many patients who see benefits report immediate relief. In one controlled clinical trial, 42 percent of patients reported reduced pain and urgency with heparin after the first treatment—double the rate of the control group. Because it has a different mechanism of action than many analgesic medications, heparin is often combined with numbing agents, such as lidocaine, in bladder instillations.

• **Lidocaine**

Lidocaine is a commonly used local numbing agent, found in everything from skin creams to injections. In cases of interstitial cystitis, instillations of lidocaine have been shown to reduce bladder pain rapidly: More than 75 percent of patients who use an instilled combination of heparin and lidocaine experience pain relief within twenty minutes. One study demonstrated that increasing the percentage of lidocaine from 1 to 2 percent raised the percentage of patients who saw improvement from 75 to 94 percent after twenty minutes of instillation. So, don't be afraid to ask for the higher dose in your treatment.

"Lidocaine is fast acting, but it's not effective for extended symptom relief."

Lidocaine is often combined with other medications so the numbing agent can rapidly reduce pain while other agents address the pain and urinary symptoms with a different method of action. This is because lidocaine is fast acting, but it's not effective for extended symptom relief: Only 30 percent of patients report that the pain reduction lasted for three days after treatment. So, if lidocaine is the sole medication in your instillation, you should be prepared to have the procedure performed twice weekly. If it's used in combination with another medication, you may see a benefit for a longer period. Lidocaine is also used in the catheterization process—the catheter can be coated in it to reduce irritation during insertion. The AUA ranks lidocaine as a second-line treatment, with an evidence ranking of a "B."

Some doctors use a similar numbing agent, Marcaine (bupivacaine), instead of lidocaine for instillations. The two drugs have the same mechanism of action, and should perform in the same manner. In other applications, Marcaine takes longer to take effect, but it has a longer period of efficacy than lidocaine—one reason some doctors work with it in a bladder cocktail. Otherwise, Marcaine should work very similarly to Lidocaine for most patients.

• Other Instillations

Some doctors include liquid PPS, a common oral medication, in bladder cocktails. This instillation has shown a limited benefit in patients: In a controlled trial, 40 percent of patients showed improvement at three months as compared to 20 percent for the placebo group. It doesn't seem to offer as much benefit as some of the other intravesical therapies, but it may have a different mechanism of action and can be worth trying in a bladder cocktail. Still, it's not recommended for use on its own in bladder instillations.

Two other instillations that have been studied are no longer suggested for use by any IC patients. The AUA recommends that patients avoid BCG (bacillus Calmette-Guérin) instillations, as little benefit was found for the treatments and more than 95 percent of patients experienced adverse events in clinical trials. Another potential treatment, resiniferatoxin (RXT), hasn't been shown to be as effective as the other instillations mentioned in this chapter, and isn't recommended, either.

"Neuromodulation is one of the most promising new medical treatments for interstitial cystitis."

Neuromodulation

Neuromodulation is one of the most promising new medical treatments for interstitial cystitis. You'll recall that the upregulation of the nervous system is one of the primary factors in the pain and urinary urgency associated with IC. During upregulation, silent nerves are activated throughout the region and the bladder signals it's full and needs to be emptied, even if you've just left the restroom. Neuromodulation artificially stimulates those nerves, which can help reset the nervous system. By retraining those nerves with outside electrical impulses, it can restore healthy function to the nerves that serve the bladder and pelvic floor. Think of nerve modulation as a pacemaker for your bladder.

There are two ways of conducting this electrical stimulation. The first is minimally invasive, but requires repeated visits to the doctor to be effective. The second requires a permanent surgical implant, which automatically stimulates the nerves throughout the day.

Percutaneous Tibial Nerve Stimulation

The less-invasive form of neuromodulation is percutaneous tibial nerve stimulation (PTNS). In this procedure, the pelvic floor nerves are targeted by an electrical impulse that's directed up the entire length of the leg: A small needle is inserted near the ankle, and the current is carried up the tibial nerve and into the pelvic floor. The tibial nerve shares some of the same roots as the bladder nerves, so, by stimulating this nerve, the procedure indirectly modulates bladder activity. This is important because the tibial nerve is much closer to the surface and far easier to access than the bladder nerves. This procedure is conducted in a doctor's office and takes about thirty minutes. The recommended course of treatment is one visit weekly for twelve consecutive weeks.

It takes time to see benefits from PTNS: There's a significant improvement between visits 6 and 12 in the clinical studies, so you'll need to commit to the full treatment course to determine how well it works for you. If it does work, a monthly maintenance visit is recommended to ensure the benefits continue.

In two major clinical trials with more than 300 overactive bladder patients, the tibial nerve procedure was shown to reduce urgency and frequency for 55 to 79 percent of patients. In contrast, the "sham" procedure, in which a needle was inserted but no electrical current applied, only helped 21 percent of the control group. Two-thirds of those who had the PTNS treatment were satisfied with the results they achieved. A three-year follow-up study of patients who had monthly maintenance visits showed that urinary frequency had dropped from twelve to nine times daily, and with one less nocturnal restroom visit each night. The machine used in this procedure is FDA-cleared as a medical device for urinary urgency and frequency, showing it has been judged to be safe and effective. However, clinical testing has focused primarily on patients with overactive bladder, and not specifically interstitial cystitis. But the same nerves and mechanisms are at work in both conditions, and many IC patients have reported the same kinds of benefits.

Percutaneous Sacral or Pudendal Nerve Stimulation

The other type of neuromodulation treatment goes right to the source: It targets the sacral or pudendal nerve endings that connect from your spinal cord to your pelvic floor. Here, the needle is inserted into the upper buttocks to stimulate the nerve roots responsible for the bladder. The goal is to implant a permanent device surgically under the skin that continually modulates these nerves.

This procedure is unique because, as a patient, you're given a test run to see whether the surgery will be beneficial before the operation. A needle is inserted into the sacral area and a low-voltage current runs through the area. The needle is taped in place for several days while doctors monitor your symptoms. If the procedure is going to be successful, you'll have significant symptom reduction within the first few days. Studies have shown that about two-thirds of patients respond positively to the initial trial.

After you know how well the device will work from the initial trial, you'll have the option to make it permanent. In clinical trials, the vast majority of patients who saw a major benefit with the trial elect to proceed with the surgery, during which a smaller version of the device is implanted to power the ongoing electrical stimulation of the nerves: A small disk, a little larger than a silver dollar, is surgically inserted beneath the skin in the upper buttock. If you're a thin person, the outline of this disk will be visible, and may even cause discomfort when sitting or lying in certain positions. For those with a little more padding, this tends to be less of an issue.

Unlike tibial nerve stimulation, sacral and pudendal nerve modulation has been tested with IC patients and the results have been published. In a 2002 study of twenty-one women, fourteen responded positively to the initial, external trial run. Of these, nearly 80 percent had the device implanted for long-term use—and those patients had very favorable results. Both daytime and nocturnal urinary frequency decreased by nearly 50 percent. Approximately two-thirds of patients saw at least moderate improvement in their urinary urgency, frequency, and pain over the course of the trial. These results confirmed those of a 2001 trial of fifteen patients with IC, in which the authors noted a 45 percent decrease in urinary frequency. Of the women in the trial procedure, 73 percent elected to proceed with the permanent implant.

The device has been FDA-cleared for use in overactive bladder since the late 1990s and has been used in nearly 200,000 patients so far. Although this technology initially focused on reducing the urinary symptoms of IC, it has had a large effect on pain, as well. In a study of ten patients with chronic pelvic pain, 60 percent reported significant improvements in their pain levels with this implantable device.

If you elect to have this procedure, take it seriously. Remember that it's surgery. You should see a physical therapist after the procedure to make sure the device isn't adhering to the surrounding tissue and that the developing scar tissue is healthy. Fortunately, the programming of the device can be adjusted remotely by the manufacturer, without requiring a second surgery. If it does stop working for you at some point, the device is usually just left in place; removal is a difficult procedure that can result in additional complications. Although this is a permanent solution, it can truly be a game changer for some patients.

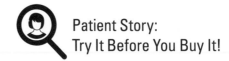

Patient Story: Try It Before You Buy It!

The unique benefit of sacral and pudendal nerve modulation is that you get to try it out before committing to permanent surgery. Typically, you'll have at least two to four days with the temporary unit to determine how your body responds. Keep a symptom log during this time to see how it works for you. Studies have shown that this technique typically helps 50 to 75 percent of patients, so you may not experience any benefit: Other patients show only a mild benefit, which may not be worth the surgery. On the other hand, if your symptoms are significantly improved with the temporary procedure, the surgery may be ideal for you.

If you're seeing a pelvic floor PT, have her evaluate you before going forward with the full procedure: Correct placement of the electrical lead is crucial, and a slight adjustment can make all the difference. For instance, a patient came to me during her temporary phase. She had major improvements in her symptoms, but something felt wrong to her. After an examination, we found that her pelvic floor was incredibly tight and spasming: The device's placement was helping her bladder symptoms but irritating her pelvic floor, which would have resulted in major problems later on. She returned to the doctor and had the placement of the lead adjusted, and her pelvic floor condition improved. Other patients have reported that the lead may irritate the sciatic nerve, which can be alleviated by a slight shift in positioning. Remember, this may be the only type of surgery you can take for a test drive—take advantage of it!

Fulguration of Hunner's Lesions

As we've discussed, a small subset of patients with interstitial cystitis have wounds within the bladder, known as Hunner's lesions. Although once thought to be central to the disease, recent studies estimate that fewer than 10 percent of patients with IC actually have these lesions. They appear primarily in older patients, often over the age of fifty, and they're identified through a cystoscopy, which many doctors perform as part of the initial diagnosis of interstitial cystitis. If these bladder ulcers are present, they can be treated by cauterizing the area either with a laser or electrocautery.

Results of these procedures have generally been good: Most patients experience relief in pain and urinary symptoms after their lesions have been cauterized. However, these ulcers often reappear and continually have to be addressed. Studies have found that patients often experience a relapse in symptoms after only a few months, though some patients experience longer periods of relief. Just be aware that they'll probably reappear and require additional treatment in the future. The AUA guidelines for interstitial cystitis consider this to be a third-line treatment, and many patients report significant benefits after having the lesions cauterized.

Hydrodistention

Hydrodistention is the process of artificially filling the bladder to capacity by injecting a liquid solution through a catheter. It is used in conjunction with most bladder procedures, including the diagnostic cystoscopy and cauterization of Hunner's lesions. These procedures are often uncomfortable and can cause symptoms to flare when the catheter is inserted into the bladder through the irritated urethra, but some patients do report an easing of symptoms immediately after a hydrodistention. At least some hydrodistentions contain the topical anesthetic lidocaine, which may explain some of the benefits experienced by patients. Generally, though, most patients are better off with an instillation that contains medication, such as a topical painkiller, rather than just a saline instillation that contains no active medication for the bladder. The AUA considers low pressure hydrodistention a third-line treatment.

Intra-Bladder BOTOX

Botulinum toxin (BTX, BOTOX) is a medication that's temporarily toxic to nerves: Regular injections over the course of several months can weaken or freeze a muscle. Best known as a cosmetic surgery agent, BTX is also used to treat muscle spasms in many different conditions, such as with migraines or cerebral palsy. In normal voiding, the bladder fills and expands. As it does so it signals the brain, prompting the need to urinate. But with interstitial cystitis, the bladder muscles are overtaxed and can spasm uncontrollably, increasing the signals sent to the brain and, therefore, the urges to urinate. In IC patients, BTX works by dampening the nerves of the muscles and allowing them to relax. A tube is inserted into the bladder to inject the detrusor muscle with the medication. By weakening the involuntary muscles of the bladder, BTX can help stop the spasms that trigger false urgency reports to the brain.

"The effects of BOTOX therapies throughout the body typically peak around two or three months after the injections and then begin to fade."

In multiple clinical trials of this newer therapy, which have been mostly based in Taiwan and Italy, BOTOX injections for IC patients have shown benefits in urinary urgency, frequency, and pain. Even when used as a therapy for patients who have tried several other treatments, most studies showed positive effects in more than half of all patients. The most recent technique has combined BOTOX injections with hydrodistention of the bladder several weeks later to optimize results. The effects of BOTOX therapies throughout the body typically peak around two or three months after the injections and then begin to fade. The best results have been seen with repeated injections of BTX, approximately every six months.

Intra-bladder BTX has recently been promoted to a fourth-line treatment by the American Urological Association because of the new research that shows it improves patient outcomes, but concerns remain about the adverse effects associated with paralyzing the muscles of the bladder. Patients who undergo this procedure have a higher risk of difficult or painful urination, because the muscles that contract to expel urine are substantially weakened. But this effect is transitory, and will wear off along with the BTX. Other patients may find that they have residual urine they're unable to void, and may be forced to self-catheterize to fully empty the bladder when the effect of the BTX is at its peak. Advances in the methods of injection have reduced this outcome, but it is still a risk that patients need to be aware of. So, if you are considering BTX, you should be willing to self-catheterize, if necessary, to remove any excess urine you're unable to release after the muscles have been relaxed; approximately 7 percent of patients had to self-catheterize at least once after receiving BTX.

The good news is the effects of this treatment are noticeable within a few weeks of the injection. Also, it's a single treatment, so you can determine whether your body responds positively to it. If it does, these injections can give you an invaluable six-month window of reduced symptoms, allowing you to work on pelvic floor physical therapy and stretching, and simply giving your bladder a chance to relax. This procedure has shown substantial benefit for many patients who haven't seen improvement with other treatments and may be a valuable option.

Bladder Removal Surgery

Bladder removal is considered a method of last resort in interstitial cystitis, and it is difficult to imagine a set of circumstances in which it would be appropriate—particularly because patients often still have pain and phantom feelings of urgency even after the bladder has been completely removed. Once it was a relatively common procedure, but the American Urological Association has relegated these surgeries to the final level of treatment, meaning that such drastic, irreversible surgery should be tried only as an absolute final option after all other treatments, therapies, and alternative approaches have been ineffective, or if the bladder has been heavily damaged by another disease.

Takeaways

- **You'll know very quickly whether bladder treatments work.** Intra-bladder medication can provide rapid pain and symptom relief for some patients. Fulguration of Hunner's lesions and intra-bladder BOTOX also give rapid feedback. Neuromodulation is one of the few surgeries you can "test drive," and you'll find out within a few days whether it will be effective for you.

- **A cocktail of different intra-bladder medications is your best bet.** All bladder medications have only been shown to work in a subset of patients. Most of the potential for side effects stems from irritation of the urethra and bladder from the procedure itself, not from the medication. Give yourself the best chance of success by using several different medications in your bladder instillations.

- **Bladder treatments are like a rest stop on the trail.** The temporary pain and symptom relief of bladder treatments give you a break, but they don't ultimately bring you much closer to your destination. Think of these periods during which your symptoms have abated as rest stops on your journey, where you can prepare for the path ahead.

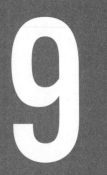

9

BEYOND THE BLADDER:

Pelvic Floor Physical Therapy for IC

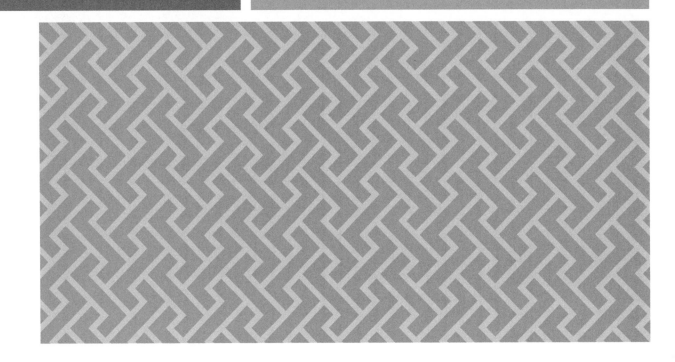

The pain and urinary symptoms of interstitial cystitis have two different sources. They can come directly from the bladder, but they can also result from musculoskeletal problems within the surrounding pelvic floor. Trigger points in the muscles, inflammation, weakness, or tightness can all create symptoms of IC. The goal of pelvic floor physical therapy, therefore, is to eliminate the portion of symptoms caused by these musculoskeletal problems in and around the pelvic floor.

With the complex interaction between the bladder and pelvic floor, a dysfunctional pelvic floor is responsible for at least some of the pain and urinary symptoms in just about every IC patient. A few patients, if they are diagnosed early on, may have relatively little pelvic floor involvement. But for many, the pelvic floor is actually the primary source of symptoms; a full, sustainable recovery has to address pelvic floor dysfunction. This chapter explains why pelvic floor physical therapy may be the most valuable treatment for your IC, how it alleviates symptoms, where to find the right physical therapist for you, and how to get the most out of your sessions.

To review, pelvic floor physical therapy is essential in disrupting the dysfunction—inflammation—pain cycle (DIP cycle; see chapter 5) in the area surrounding the bladder. Tight and knotted muscles are unable to function properly and contribute to your IC symptoms; physical therapy addresses these problems at the source to restore normal function. IC causes inflammation to stagnate in the pelvic region; physical therapy releases the trapped swelling and increases blood flow to sweep it away. Trigger points refer pain to the bladder, urethra, and throughout the pelvic region; physical therapy works to systematically release these hypersensitive spots. Pelvic floor physical therapy, then, is the only treatment that can address all three aspects of the DIP cycle: dysfunction, inflammation, and pain.

Clinical Evidence for Pelvic Floor Physical Therapy in IC

Pelvic floor physical therapy is one of the most-proven treatments for interstitial cystitis. It is the only treatment for IC given an evidence grade of "A" by the American Urological Association guidelines, which recommends it in the first line of medical treatment. Many clinical trials have been conducted to evaluate pelvic floor physical therapy for interstitial cystitis, as well as others for chronic pelvic pain conditions. And the results are consistently positive. The majority of patients improve significantly with physical therapy, with little risk of adverse events.

One of the earliest physical therapy studies evaluated IC patients who had struggled with the condition for an average of fourteen years. Conducted in San Francisco and published in 2001, this study revolutionized IC treatment. These were patients who had tried just about everything else without finding relief. But with just one or two treatments a week for eight to twelve weeks, 70 percent of patients treated reported more than a 50 percent improvement in their symptoms.

It's remarkable that patients who had been struggling with their condition for decades without success saw such dramatic improvement in less than three months. The research also tried to quantify how much pelvic floor physical therapy could release muscular tension, and found that stress in the pelvic floor decreased by 65 percent for these IC patients.

Several years later these results were confirmed by a similar study. Over the course of six treatments, the use of intravaginal physical therapy led to improvements in pain, urgency, and frequency in 90 percent of women involved. The patients showed substantial improvement in control over their pelvic floor muscles, as well. Another trial evaluated physical therapy over the course of just five weeks. With two treatments a week, in a little more than a month patients saw statistically significant improvements in pain, urgency, frequency, and their mental and physical quality of life.

The gold standard for testing pelvic floor physical therapy in interstitial cystitis is a pair of studies published in 2009 and 2012. Many of the top institutions in the country—including Stanford, University of Michigan, University of Pennsylvania, Loyola University, the Cleveland Clinic, and the University of California, San Diego—collaborated with the National Institutes of Health to study pelvic floor physical therapy as a treatment for interstitial cystitis.

Unlike other IC studies, these were randomized and controlled, with the control group receiving a standard therapeutic massage. The initial study used six different sites to ensure the results weren't due to a single exceptional therapist. Each patient received treatment for one hour over the course of ten weekly treatments.

The results were striking. In the first study, patients showed significant benefits in pain, urgency, frequency, overall symptom scores, and sexual function after just ten weeks of treatment, and the treatments were effective for both men and women.

IMPROVEMENTS WITH 10 WEEKS OF PHYSICAL THERAPY

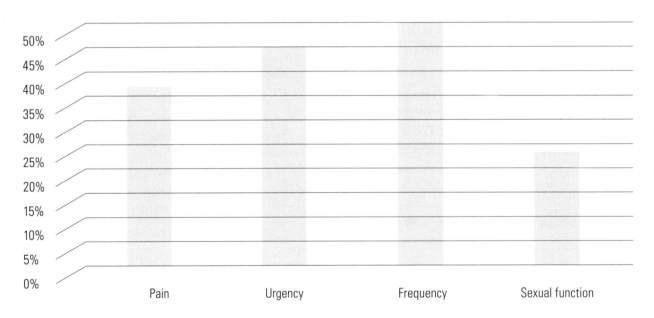

Average improvement in IC symptoms with ten sessions of physical therapy.
Source: FitzGerald, M., R. Anderson, J. Potts, et al. "Randomized Multicenter Feasibility Trial of Myosfascial Physical Therapy for Treatment of Urologic Chronic Pelvic Pain Syndrome," *The Journal of Urology* 182, no. 2 (June 2009): 570–80.

These benefits for IC were confirmed by many of the same researchers in a large, well-designed follow-up study. Eleven sites and more than eighty IC patients were evaluated, and the authors, again, confirmed that nearly 90 percent of patients saw a benefit from the treatment, with large reductions in pain and improvements in urinary symptoms. Significant reductions in pain, urgency, and frequency were noted in the treatment group as compared to those in the control group, and the women in the group reported a substantial improvement in sexual function, as well. In quality of life questionnaires, the patients reported benefits in both their physical and mental status from physical therapy.

Pelvic Floor Physical Therapy for Chronic Prostatitis

You might remember, especially if you're male, we discussed chronic prostatitis in chapter 4. We noted that it's certainly interrelated with IC, and might even be the same condition. The authors of the multisite NIH study also evaluated chronic prostatitis patients, using the same physical therapy techniques. The response was nearly identical between the IC group and chronic prostatitis: Both groups showed similar reductions in pain, urinary symptoms, and overall symptoms. Men diagnosed with chronic prostatitis actually saw even more benefit from pelvic floor physical therapy than those with an IC diagnosis.

Again, regardless of how chronic prostatitis and IC end up being classified—whether as a single condition or two interrelated ones—IC treatments are consistently shown to be effective for men diagnosed with chronic prostatitis.

PATIENT SYMPTOM SUMMARY

	Interstitial cystitis	Chronic prostatitis
Reduction in pain	37 percent	43 percent
Improvement in urinary symptoms	45 percent	44 percent
IC symptom index	35 percent	47 percent
Improvement in sexual function	39 percent	57 percent

Percent of improvement in symptoms with pelvic floor physical therapy in both IC and chronic prostatitis.
Source: FitzGerald, M., C. Payne, E. Lukacz, et al. "Randomized Multicenter Clinical Trial of Myofascial Physical Therapy in Women with Interstitial Cystitis/Painful Bladder Syndrome (IC/PBS) and Pelvic Floor Tenderness," *The Journal of Urology* 187, no. 6 (June 2012): 2113–18.

External Physical Therapy

The external component of pelvic floor physical therapy focuses primarily on the muscles and ligaments that attach directly to your pelvic floor and contribute to IC symptoms. As discussed in chapter 5, all muscles lead to the bony pelvis: Your abdominal muscles, lower back muscles, hamstrings, quads, glutes, and hip flexors all attach there. Any or all of these muscles can place tension on the pelvic floor. And tighter muscles on one side versus the other can create a torque on the pelvis. This may not seem like a big deal, but it is. This twisting force can be so pronounced that you can actually see it: In many people, one hip is visibly higher or one leg has a longer stride than the other. The same thing can happen to the abdomen. If the abdominal muscles are tight, the entire pelvis will be tilted in that direction. This external force creates problems for the pelvis, and for the other attached muscles.

The focus of the external physical therapy is to ensure that all muscles are in balance, and aren't creating an outside force on the pelvic floor. To achieve this, your PT can address a muscle that's too tight and is pulling harder on the pelvis than it should, or strengthen a muscle that's too weak to hold up its end of the bargain. Hip or low back pain may also be straining your pelvis, and should be addressed in physical therapy.

Physical therapy can loosen tight or knotted muscles. By massaging out knots or trigger points, the entire muscle can relax and return to normal function. The hamstrings, glutes, lower back, and abdominal muscles are often very tight in interstitial cystitis patients. Trigger points in these muscles can refer pain into the pelvis and bladder, so releasing the tension from these muscles can ease many of the symptoms associated with IC.

The other way to affect the pelvic floor is by strengthening muscles that have atrophied or become too weak. The human body is incredible in the way it compensates for a muscle group that isn't pulling its weight. However, if one muscle group is significantly weaker than the others that attach to the pelvis, the pelvis can be pulled away from the weak muscle and cause problems. Your therapist will help you identify the weak muscles and develop a customized strengthening program for them.

Patients often also carry tension in the complex series of connective tissue underneath the skin and above the muscles, known as the fascia. Inflammation often gets trapped in this area, causing the skin to stick to the muscles underneath and become painful to the touch. The abdominal area above the bladder, hamstrings, and inner thighs is the area most affected. This lingering inflammation causes tightness in the muscles beneath and decreases blood flow, creating dysfunction that feeds back into bladder symptoms. The medical term for this is *subcutaneous panniculosis*. A physical therapist can release this tension through a process called myofascial release, which uses smooth, gliding strokes to free the skin and restore blood flow to the region to remove the remnants of inflammation. The skin will be able to move freely again, instead of adhering to the muscles underneath and reinforcing painful trigger points. Releasing the tension in the fascia can have a direct and profound impact on IC symptoms.

 fas·ci·a (noun):
Connective tissue found underneath the skin throughout the body that separates the skin from the muscles underneath and plays an important role in blood flow and the inflammatory response.

Internal Physical Therapy

Many important muscles within the pelvic floor can only be reached internally, but they can be treated the same way as muscles that are externally accessible. Relaxing too-tight internal muscles and releasing trigger points releases tension in the pelvic floor and restores healthy function to the bladder. For women, there are two ways to reach the internal pelvic floor muscles: either vaginally or rectally. For men, the rectal option is the sole choice. In the same way she works with muscles on the outside of the body, your physical therapist will search for trigger points that tighten the muscles and will work to release them by placing gentle pressure on them until they release.

In your initial examination, your physical therapist will try to reproduce your IC symptoms as she works on your pelvic floor. My patients are always shocked to realize that the symptoms they thought were bladder related actually stem from strained pelvic muscles. It's true: A trigger point in the pelvic floor can reproduce the urgent need to urinate. And suprapubic, hip, or lower back pain can be recreated by gently pressing on these tight internal muscles. Though it may be uncomfortable at first, the ability to reproduce these symptoms is actually a good thing. It confirms at least some of your pain and urgency originates from the pelvic floor muscles, which proves it can be treated to provide relief.

In interstitial cystitis patients, the small muscles that control the urethra are often among the most sensitive—overworked, angry, and strained. These muscles often cause the urinary urgency and frequency considered to be bladder symptoms. As these trigger points are released, the urinary symptoms begin to ease. In clinical trials with IC patients, ten sessions of physical therapy reduced urinary urgency by 40 percent and cut trips to the bathroom in half.

Another important aspect of internal physical therapy is reducing or preventing the pain with sex that often accompanies IC. Dyspareunia (painful intercourse) is extremely common with interstitial cystitis, generally manifesting as pain with intercourse for women or pain after ejaculation for men. This is because the muscles that control sexual arousal and orgasm are located within the pelvic floor, and are also knotted and dysfunctional. Your pelvic floor therapist can locate these muscles and release the trigger points within them, working to restore healthy, pain-free sexual function.

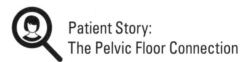 Patient Story:
The Pelvic Floor Connection

Amanda came into the clinic because her urogynecologist referred her to pelvic floor physical therapy for her interstitial cystitis. She had classic IC symptoms—suprapubic discomfort and urinary urgency and frequency. During her session, she mentioned she was also seeing an orthopedic PT because of pain in her hip, but was about to stop because it wasn't helping.

Just a few minutes later, during her initial examination, we found an internal trigger point that reproduced both her urgent need to urinate and the exact feeling of her hip pain! She hadn't been improving with traditional physical therapy because the problem wasn't in her hip—it was based in her pelvic floor. Releasing that trigger point eliminated most of her urinary symptoms, as well as the hip pain she had been dealing with for months.

Treatment Milestones with Physical Therapy

All patients want to know what to expect from pelvic floor physical therapy. Studies on PT tend to allow at least ten visits before they assess how well the treatment is working—but it's natural to want assurances about when you'll start seeing improvement, how much improvement to expect, and when you can decrease visits to the clinic and rely on self-care instead. Ultimately, the answers depend on each individual. You may see fantastic results almost immediately, within the first few sessions, while others may take several months. If you've been struggling with undiagnosed or untreated IC for years, it may take even longer to reverse the persistent dysfunction.

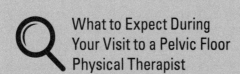

What to Expect During Your Visit to a Pelvic Floor Physical Therapist

- Ideally, 45 to 60 minutes of hands-on PT
- Both internal and external work in every session
- No use (or limited use) of physical therapy aides
- The ability to refer to other practitioners for medical management
- No Kegel exercises
- Instruction in a specific self-care home program

Your results depend on how long you've had the condition and how much time you're willing to spend on self-care techniques when you aren't at the PT clinic.

Despite individual variability, these signposts ensure you're on the road to recovery with your physical therapist.

- On your first visit, the physical therapist should be able to reproduce some of your symptoms, with either internal or external trigger point work or myofascial release. Remember, it's a good thing if a PT is able to reproduce your IC symptoms: It means there's an identifiable musculoskeletal component to your condition that can be treated and eliminated.

- You should also see a change of some sort within the first four to six sessions. This may not be a dramatic, universal improvement. Sometimes alleviating one trouble spot within the pelvic floor uncovers a new area that needs attention, so the symptoms may shift. For example, you might notice a decrease in pain but a temporary increase in frequency. Or, you may have soreness, or even a flare of symptoms, immediately after a treatment. But this is still a positive change—a normal part of the healing process.

However, if you don't notice any substantial differences after your first six visits, you may need to reevaluate your treatment plan with your therapist. Assess whether you've been doing your part by completing home exercises or stretching assigned by your physical therapist, and whether there might be any outside factors preventing you from improving.

Increasing Activities with Physical Therapy

One of the biggest advantages of pelvic floor physical therapy is that it allows you to regain aspects of your life you may have abandoned because of your symptoms. With the help of your PT, you can add activities back into your life: The physical therapy can keep your symptoms at a manageable level even as you increase your activity.

This can be very helpful as you settle back into an exercise routine, for example. The first few times you exercise after a period of inactivity can be difficult, and may put additional strain on the pelvic floor. But your PT can help keep your pelvic floor healthy as you begin a new exercise program and gradually increase its intensity. Or, you may experience setbacks when returning to work after a leave of absence: Sitting places additional stress on the pelvic floor, so returning to a desk job can cause symptoms to flare again. You can minimize these flares and keep trigger points from contributing to your symptoms by working with a physical therapist as you transition back into your job.

Finding a Great Pelvic Floor Physical Therapist

The field of pelvic floor physical therapy is relatively new and is growing rapidly. Training standards vary widely between therapists, and it can be difficult to find a great pelvic floor PT. Just as you would with any healthcare practitioner, don't be afraid to ask questions about experience and qualifications. After all, your PT is likely the professional with whom you will interact the most. She can guide your care, recommend local specialists to help with the medical management, and teach you about your pelvic floor and how to keep it healthy. So, selecting your physical therapist is an important decision.

When doing research in this regard, the first questions to ask are about credentials and years of experience. There is a board certification for a specialty in this field, known as a Women's Clinical Specialist (WCS). A therapist with this certification is your best bet (even if you are a man, despite the certification name), because these specialists are extensively trained in all kinds of pelvic floor dysfunction. This certification requires extensive education, several years of full-time experience with pelvic floor patients, passing an exhaustive written test, and completing a case study on a pelvic floor patient. It's a relatively rare specialty, and you may have difficulty finding a local therapist with a WCS certification. There are currently fewer than 300 of these specialists in the United States.

If there's no WCS-certified therapist near you, ask about years of experience with pelvic floor patients. Ideally, you want to know your therapist has been working with patients like you for at least several years. If you are seeing someone new to the field, she should be working regularly with an experienced mentor. Feel free to ask your therapist about their continuing education. Because the pelvic floor is rarely addressed in PT school, most training comes from intensive continuing education courses after graduation. Your PT should have attended several of these courses. Don't worry about asking questions. Any good physical therapist will be happy to discuss her training and experience with you. If not, she may not be the right person to work with.

You should also ask about how much hands-on time you'll receive with your PT during the appointment. In general, the longer the treatment session, the better. An hour-long session with your therapist ensures there's time to address both internal and external aspects of treatment. And, the therapist should be dedicated to manual therapy, with external and internal work a part of each visit. Make sure you only count time with the physical therapist, not with an aide who may help with exercises or stretching.

 ## To Kegel or Not to Kegel?

With IC, it's not even a question—**you should not be doing Kegel exercises.** A Kegel is a deliberate contraction or tightening of your pelvic floor muscles. These exercises are often recommended for everything from reducing incontinence to improving your sex life. Kegel exercises do have a place, particularly for patients with incontinence or prolapse, whose dysfunction stems from a weak pelvic floor. However, for IC they are one of the worst things you can do. If you've tried Kegel exercises and experienced an increase in symptoms, it's not just your imagination.

For nearly all IC patients, your pelvic floor is already too tight. The challenge is to relax it, not tighten it further. Pelvic floor physical therapy focuses on reducing the tension and trigger points within the pelvic floor. The only time adding Kegel exercises to your treatment plan might be appropriate is near the end, after your pelvic floor is mostly clear of trigger points and dysfunction. Under the close supervision of your pelvic floor PT, Kegels may be added as part of your core strengthening program or to address another pelvic floor problem, such as incontinence or prolapse. Do not perform Kegels without the recommendation of a qualified PT.

Checklist to Finding the Right PT for You

- If at all possible, look for a clinic that specializes in pelvic floor physical therapy.
- Look for the Women's Clinical Specialist (WCS) credential, even if you're male; a PT with this credential can treat both men and women.
- If there is no one with the WCS credential near you, look for a practitioner with several years' experience with pelvic floor patients.
- Most pelvic floor education for PTs comes after they've left school and from intensive continuing education courses. Your PT should have attended several of these courses.
- Ask how much time you'll receive with your PT; in general, the longer the treatment session, the better. (Make sure you count only time with the PT, not an aide.)
- If, after four to six visits, there's been no improvement, consider re-evaluating your options for PT.

If at all possible, look for a clinic that specializes in pelvic floor physical therapy. It's best to work with a medical professional who has chosen to work with patients like you. As awareness of the benefits of pelvic floor therapy increase, some large clinics are adding a single therapist with limited experience in pelvic floor therapy to attract additional patients. Although it's certainly possible for these therapists to be well qualified, it's also possible that they've taken only a single weekend course on the subject, and aren't truly specialists in the field. If you aren't noticing a change or improvement in symptoms after your first four to six visits, don't be afraid to reevaluate your options for physical therapy.

As with medical doctors, you may not be able to find a true specialist in your local area. If that's the case, it can be helpful to make a special trip to visit a top-notch pelvic floor physical therapist. Even a single visit can give you a great deal of clarity about your condition and what will help it. Plus, a highly respected clinic may be able to give you a good recommendation for a local physical therapist near you. Even if your local PT doesn't have as much experience, the therapist in the specialty clinic can help you develop a treatment plan and guide your care. Take advantage of twenty-first-century communication: call, email, Skype, or travel to get the best advice and care that you can. Most well-known pelvic floor specialists will have a program for out-of-town patients. The expert you meet should also be able to coordinate care with your hometown physical therapist, or provide a detailed care plan that another therapist can help you follow.

Frequently Asked Questions about IC and Pelvic Floor Physical Therapy

Why is this happening to me all of a sudden?
Typically, pelvic floor dysfunction has been present for years before a patient visits a physical therapist. Perhaps symptoms were minor, at such a low level you didn't think anything of it. You may have taken a few more bathroom stops than your friends, experienced occasional pain during sex, or felt a twinge in your stomach with a full bladder.

What is the reason for my pelvic floor dysfunction?
Interstitial cystitis automatically triggers pelvic floor dysfunction. This may be exacerbated by other causes—a fall on your tailbone, pelvic surgery, or childbirth all can cause trauma to the pelvic region and spark a chain reaction of pelvic floor problems. It's likely that a combination of factors is responsible. Regardless of the root cause, true healing from IC requires addressing and fixing the pelvic floor component of your symptoms.

How long until I get better?
Pelvic floor issues are incredibly complex, and vary from patient to patient. Someone just diagnosed with IC and who felt symptoms only recently can't be compared to someone struggling with the condition for decades without addressing the pelvic floor.

If your physical therapist can recreate any of your urinary or pain symptoms by touching a muscle in your pelvic floor, then it's something that can be treated. You should notice a difference in about four to six visits and then steady improvement in symptoms and your level of daily functioning.

Muscle-Relaxant Suppositories for the Pelvic Floor

Some physicians have prescribed muscle relaxants as suppositories. Most muscle relaxants affect the central nervous system, not the local tissue, by inhibiting receptors in the brain and spinal cord. About the same amount of medication enters the bloodstream whether you take a muscle relaxant orally or as a suppository, so a suppository isn't useless. But it's obviously less convenient to take medication rectally or vaginally, and having to hold the suppository in place until it dissolves can irritate the pelvic floor.

Muscle relaxants can be a great complement to physical therapy. They can prevent some of the rebound effect in which a muscle released by the physical therapist tightens up again after treatment. By allowing you to maintain the gains of a PT session, a muscle relaxant can speed recovery. Talk to your doctor about which method of delivery is best for you.

Why didn't my doctor know about pelvic floor physical therapy? Many patients find out about pelvic floor physical therapy on their own. When they get better with PT, they often express frustration that their medical practitioners didn't recommend it earlier. Unfortunately, doctors are often unaware of how much pelvic floor dysfunction contributes to IC symptoms. It's entirely possible that your doctor went through medical school, several years of residency, and even specialty training in the field while receiving perhaps, a single hourlong lecture on pelvic floor anatomy. Musculoskeletal problems within the pelvic floor are just not on the radar for most doctors—though with additional research and education in the field, we hope that will change.

Medical Treatment and Pelvic Floor Physical Therapy

Traditional medical treatment can complement physical therapy, allowing you to improve as rapidly as possible. As we've discussed, oral medications and bladder treatments can reduce symptoms. That helps break the DIP (dysfunction–inflammation–pain) cycle and allows the physical therapist to do more work without irritating or flaring symptoms. Reducing pain and urinary symptoms allows you to participate more actively in your treatment with a self-care program to maintain the advances you make during physical therapy between visits. Any medical treatment that reduces pain and inflammation will have a positive effect on your progress. There are also medical treatments specifically designed to augment physical therapy.

Suppositories

Suppositories are medications inserted into the vagina or rectum to deliver medication directly to the pelvic floor. As with bladder instillations, the major benefit is that the medicine is applied directly to the tissue that needs it. Suppositories are designed to dissolve after they have been inserted, where they are absorbed through the walls of the vagina or rectum into the pelvic floor and bloodstream.

Almost all information regarding the use of suppositories for relieving pain and symptoms is anecdotal and not strongly supported with clinical trials. When considering whether to try a suppository or not, make sure the drug is one that works topically on the tissues to which it is applied. Many pain medications or muscle relaxants work on nerves in the brain and spinal cord, not at the place where they're applied: In these cases, a suppository may be of no benefit over oral administration.

Patients often report that the most successful suppositories contain lidocaine or another numbing agent. These drugs work directly on the muscles and nerves to which they are applied to ease pain. However, lidocaine and other numbing agents can also be irritating to the tissues of the vagina or rectum, and should be used with caution. Some patients report that lidocaine can cause a burning sensation, and overuse can dry out the lining of the vagina or rectum. It's not a long-term solution, but it can be helpful, especially when you're just starting your pelvic floor physical therapy.

There are several ways to get the most out of your suppository prescription. If you're keeping a symptom log or being mindful of your body, you should be familiar with the times of day at which you feel best—and worst. Maybe you're generally better in the mornings, but your symptoms increase in the afternoon, or vice versa. It can be helpful to use the suppository when symptoms worsen, to press the reset button, so to speak, on your pain.

You can also use a numbing agent suppository before or after pelvic floor physical therapy to augment your treatment. If you are just starting out with physical therapy and are highly sensitive, it can sometimes be helpful to use the suppository an hour prior to your treatment session. It will deaden the sensation and help the pelvic floor relax naturally, which can make the therapy more effective. Or, after treatment, you may feel sore or sensitive from having those tight muscles worked on; using a suppository at that point can prevent symptoms from flaring. Your doctor or physical therapist can give you detailed advice on how and when to use your suppository.

We've also discussed the role of oral muscle relaxants as a component of treatment. A systemic muscle relaxant can be helpful during physical therapy: It can prevent some of the rebound effect, in which a muscle released by the physical therapist tightens up again after treatment. More than 90 percent of patients who combined an oral muscle relaxant with pelvic floor physical therapy saw improvements in their pelvic dysfunction.

Trigger Point Injections for the Pelvic Floor

As we've learned, trigger points are tender areas in which the muscle is inflamed and in spasm, and that can refer pain throughout the pelvic region. Physical therapy focuses on releasing these knotted muscles to eliminate the symptoms they cause. With trigger points too stubborn or painful to respond well to physical therapy, it can help to inject medication directly into the muscle to encourage it to release. These trigger point injections are usually performed by a urogynecologist. They can contain an anesthetic, such as lidocaine, and often include a corticosteroid to reduce inflammation. These injections act rapidly, and typically last for at least three days and up to one week.

Nerve Blocks as Clues to Your IC

You can learn a lot about your interstitial cystitis from a nerve block. Here's what it can tell you:

- If it's immediately and drastically effective in reducing a symptom, then that symptom is likely due to an irritated nerve.
- If it allows your pelvic floor to relax and your next physical therapy treatment gives much more relief than usual, then many of your symptoms are related to tight muscles in the pelvic floor.
- If the nerve block doesn't help a given symptom much at all, which occurs most commonly with suprapubic pain or direct bladder pain, it indicates pelvic floor muscles and nerves are not the main causes of that particular symptom.

Trigger point injections are most effective when used to complement physical therapy. By numbing a major trigger point, they allow the physical therapist to work more freely on the surrounding muscles. Without pelvic floor physical therapy, the trigger points will simply return after the injection. Typically, you should visit your physical therapist within twenty-four hours after your trigger point injection. She'll be able to work on the area, now that it's less tender, and help the muscle relax. These injections are usually administered once per week for six consecutive weeks, with each injection followed immediately by a physical therapy appointment. Your physical therapist can map out your injection sites, so the doctor can target the biggest problems within the pelvic floor.

One concern that doctors often express to my patients is that the effect of these injections is limited: Pain and inflammation in the muscle will only be reduced for a maximum of one week after the procedure. However, this can be a very important way to break the DIP cycle. By reducing pain and inflammation, and by having your physical therapist address the dysfunction during the window of opportunity provided by the injection, all major points of that feedback loop can be addressed.

Here's where there is a gender difference in treatment: It is much easier to access the trigger points in women with these injections. That's why trigger point injections work best in female patients with specific, stubborn tender areas. After being evaluated by a physical therapist and beginning treatment, you'll learn whether there is a widespread problem, or if the majority of the issues stem from stubborn trigger points in just a few muscles. If the problem is discrete, and the trigger point injections can target those muscles, they can be very effective. If the trigger points are widespread—or if you're a man—the next option is generally a nerve block.

Nerve Blocks

Nerve blocks work similarly to trigger point injections, but the medication targets the nerve rather than the muscle tissue. A major advantage of nerve blocks is they are able to affect a wider area of the pelvic floor. If the dysfunction or pain stems from too many muscles to address with trigger point injections, a nerve block may be a better choice.

Your doctor and PT can help you decide how far up the nerve you want to try the nerve block—the higher up the nerve or spine you go, the more areas affected by the treatment. Depending on the point at which your symptoms originate, you can move the block to ensure your problem areas are included. The nerve block can be helpful in two different ways: If a symptom is caused by an irritated nerve—which often happens in a tight pelvic floor—the nerve block will immediately provide great relief. And, numbing the nerves through the pelvic floor can also help relax the area, and, with pelvic floor physical therapy, the tight pelvic floor muscles can be released. Nerve blocks serve to break the DIP cycle and may allow enough relief for physical therapy to be more effective.

Because the objective is to block nerve sensation in the pelvic floor, a nerve block can have some side effects. Constipation and stomach issues can occur, mostly because the pelvic floor is struggling with its normal task of eliminating waste. Urinary incontinence can occur, too, if the block affects the nerves that regulate urination. Occasionally, the medication will interact with the sciatic nerve that runs through the region and controls the legs, which can lead to difficulties in walking and movement for a short time after the injection. All these side effects are temporary and will only last until the nerve block wears off in a few days.

"BOTOX is a more aggressive option for patients: It requires a nerve block and should be tried only after trigger point injections have been attempted."

BOTOX to the Pelvic Floor

BOTOX (BTX-A) is a more powerful, longer-lasting form of trigger point injection that can be an option if standard trigger point injections do not give the necessary relief. BOTOX is applied in the same manner as trigger point injections, and is also difficult to use in male patients. However, instead of injecting only a few trigger points, BOTOX requires the delivery of substantially more medication to the muscles: Injections are conducted at dozens of spots within the pelvic floor. This procedure is quite painful, and is only administered after a nerve block, which minimizes the pain. Some patients even opt for a general anesthetic for the procedure.

So why would anyone go through the ordeal of BOTOX injections? Well, the primary benefit is that they last for three to four months, instead of three days for a standard trigger point injection. If you experienced good results with trigger point injections but want the effect to last substantially longer, BOTOX may be a valuable option. This approach is also much broader than the trigger point procedures, and so may be more appropriate if multiple muscle groups are causing issues within the pelvic floor.

BOTOX to the pelvic floor is never the first procedure that's recommended, and is usually only considered after both trigger point injections and nerve blocks have been tried. If you have experienced a lot of short-term benefit from trigger point injections but the knots re-form after the medication wears off, BOTOX may be a good choice for you. It extends the impact of a trigger point injection for several months, allowing you to reset the muscle memory of the pelvic floor and providing a sustained period of relief.

Unlike trigger point injections, which take effect immediately, it takes time for BOTOX to build to its peak level of impact—several weeks can pass before the neurotoxin reaches full effect. And most patients experience a short-term spike in pain and symptoms after the procedure, as the invasive injections flare the pelvic floor. This should dissipate as the BOTOX begins to take hold, though, and the numbing effect can then be at optimum level for several months.

However, patients should use caution when considering BOTOX therapy if they have untreated lower back pain or hip pain, because a weakened pelvic floor can put more orthopedic strain on the lower back. Also, be very careful when trying BOTOX if you have already had any problems with urinary incontinence, urinary retention, or constipation: These are common side effects of BOTOX treatment, so these symptoms may be exacerbated.

As you'd expect, side effects of the procedure (if present) also last for quite a long time. Incontinence, constipation, and numbness in the region can persist for as long as the BOTOX is effective. So, BOTOX is a more aggressive option for patients: It requires a nerve block and should be tried only after trigger point injections have been attempted. However, in some patients, these injections can be an important tool for breaking the DIP cycle and providing an extended period of relief.

Takeaways

- **Pelvic floor physical therapy is the single most effective treatment for interstitial cystitis.** Most patients see significant improvements in symptoms within three months of treatment. Make sure you've found the best possible therapist in your area, and commit to at least three months of PT. Be consistent about following the self-care routine your therapist recommends.

- **Full symptom relief can't be achieved by focusing solely on the bladder.** Many of your IC symptoms are directly related to the pelvic floor. Your PT should be able to reproduce some of your symptoms in an initial evaluation: If they are emanating from the pelvic floor, releasing the muscle trigger points and preventing additional nerve irritation will reduce your symptoms.

- **Your pelvic floor physical therapist can be an important guide on your IC journey.** Your PT will work more closely with you than any other medical practitioner. Choose your physical therapist wisely: She can often recommend other knowledgeable doctors, pain-management physicians, and specialists, and can offer advice on other treatments.

10

PUT YOURSELF FIRST:

Self-Care for IC

At the end of the day, success in reducing your interstitial cystitis symptoms and regaining your life depends on you. And, for better or worse, the amount of time you're able to devote to caring for yourself will play a major role in your improvement. Following a self-care program at home can help restore normal function to the pelvic floor in the same way that physical therapy can. The three main techniques to address in your self-care program are:

1. Stretching
2. Fascial release
3. Trigger point release

This chapter shows you how.

Stretching elongates tight muscles, increasing their range of motion and returning them to optimal length. It reduces or prevents trigger points from forming. Relieving the strain of tight muscles eliminates the tension on your pelvis and allows it to function properly. You'll focus on the muscles around the pelvis—the hamstrings, inner thighs, and abdominal muscles. It is also possible to stretch and loosen the pelvic floor directly.

Fascial release works to ensure the connective tissue directly underneath your skin is healthy: Inflammation can accumulate in this space, reducing blood flow to the region, and causing pain and urinary symptoms. IC patients often find that the fascia around the abdomen, hamstrings, and inner thighs is inflamed and tender. The fascia can adhere to the trigger points in the muscle below and needs to be cleared before the knot can be released.

Trigger points can be released directly with the application of gentle, sustained pressure. This relieves a major source of IC symptoms and gets the muscles in and around the pelvic floor working properly again. These three techniques can substantially reduce IC symptoms, especially as a complement to physical therapy.

Stretching

Most people tend to think of stretching as working toward increased flexibility. Elite athletes and weekend warriors stretch before games to improve performance and prevent injury. But gaining flexibility is only a small fraction of what stretching is about. For those of us who aren't professional athletes, stretching is simply about relaxing tight, tense muscles.

When you have IC, all the muscles and tissue surrounding the pelvic floor tighten up, instinctively trying to protect the bladder and pelvic floor. Even though they're just trying to help, this muscular tightness actually amplifies and contributes to the pain and urinary symptoms you experience.

For you, stretching is about giving your body permission to relax and let go of the stress you're carrying in the pelvic area. Your goal isn't to improve your flexibility. That'll happen naturally, so don't measure your progress based on whether you can touch your toes. Instead, your goal is to give your bladder a calm place to rest, reducing the pain and urinary symptoms of interstitial cystitis.

Hot Baths

Taking a bath isn't technically a form of stretching, but it provides some of the same benefits. Many patients report their symptoms ease with a long, hot bath. That's because the extended exposure to warmth allows muscles to relax and lengthen, and can actually relieve knots and tight spots within the muscles. Heat also draws blood to the surface of your skin and muscles (which is why your skin has that rosy look after being immersed in warm water). That's a good thing if you have IC—facilitating blood flow through the area can help remove built-up inflammation trapped in those tight, tense areas. Some patients like taking baths to warm the muscles before stretching, since it tends to increase muscle elasticity.

A warm bath is also an inherently calming experience for many people. It's a signal that you can completely unwind. This can help your nervous system relax, and can begin to reverse the upregulation amplifying your symptoms. Many patients will also use bath salts or aromatherapy while soaking. While there's no proven medical benefit to these complements, anything that enhances your bath experience or soothes you—including quiet music, candles, or meditation tapes—is a good thing. Do whatever you enjoy to make the bath your own private sanctuary.

Deep Breathing

Categorizing breathing as a stretch may seem odd. But the vast majority of our breathing is shallow breathing, involving only the chest. And our brains naturally associate these quick, shallow breaths with danger or anxiety, which can further upregulate the nervous system. This kind of chest breathing doesn't involve the abdominal muscles or the pelvic floor.

Deep breathing, on the other hand, comes from the belly. It relaxes the pelvic floor, calms the nervous system, and reduces stress. To practice, start by lying on your back, with your hands gently resting on your lower stomach. Your chest should remain still as your belly fills and expands. Breathe in for at least three seconds, filling your lungs completely. Hold it for a moment before you exhale: Your exhalations should be even slower than your inhalations. Pay attention to the breath and visualize the stress leaving your body with each exhale. This may feel foreign at first, but, after just seven deep breaths, you'll feel calmer, more mentally sharp, and refreshed.

Once you master deep breathing, you can—and should—do it all the time. Set aside some time each day to concentrate on your breathing. Some of my patients do their breathing exercises in the shower, which is already a warm, relaxing setting. Or, you can practice in the car on the way to work, at lunch, or before or after a stressful event. There's no such thing as too much deep breathing. Some patients set an hourly alarm to remind themselves to pay attention to their breathing—and with good reason: Even with just a few deep breaths in a row, you'll feel the pelvic floor relax, the ribcage open, and stress leave your body. It can make a huge difference. Plus, as you practice, your unconscious breathing will deepen, working for your benefit throughout the day.

Practice deep breathing while you do your other stretching and self-care exercises. When stretching, try to synchronize your movements with your exhales. And when you're doing self-massage and trigger point release, keep your breathing slow, deep, and steady. As simple as it is, deep breathing is one of the most important—and certainly the easiest—things you can do to take care of yourself.

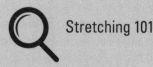

Stretching 101

Here's a crash course in safe, effective stretching. Follow these simple guidelines:

- **Discomfort is okay; pain isn't.** When stretching a tight muscle, you'll probably feel a twinge of discomfort. That's okay, but being in pain while stretching is not. If you feel pain, ease back until the stretch stops hurting. Allow your body to relax and gradually work to lengthen the stretch.

- **Avoid numbness or tingling.** When we stretch, we're working on the body's muscles. But numbness or tingling during stretching means you're actually stretching a nerve. That's the last thing you want to do! The nerves are already irritated and tender, and stretching them to the point at which they tingle is only going to make the muscles tighter.

- **Stretch until the first resistance, and no farther.** Tune in to your body when you stretch; notice when your body first resists a movement. Hold the stretch there and your muscles will gradually relax and release, allowing you to go farther. Don't try to power through that initial resistance and stretch beyond it. Doing so is counterproductive because it causes your muscles to tense.

- **Breathe and visualize.** Stretching is a great time to work on your breathing. You should breathe through your belly, using your diaphragm, and taking long, slow, controlled breaths. While stretching, try to visualize the release of tension from the muscle you're working on. For example, some of my patients imagine their muscles as melting butter while they stretch.

- **Gain without pain.** You already know that you should stop stretching if the muscle you are working hurts. But pay attention to the rest of your body, too. If you're feeling pain anywhere else during your stretching, stop. There's almost always another way to stretch the muscle that won't hurt the affected area; a physical therapist can show you how.

- **Hold each stretch for at least one minute.** Your body carries a lot of tension in your muscles, and it won't disappear immediately. A long, gradual stretch is much better than a short, intense one. Get comfortable in these positions, relax into the stretch, and you'll see much better results than if you try to blaze through your routine. You can certainly spend more time in each position, and many patients will relax into a stretch for five minutes or more at a time.

Relaxing the Pelvic Floor

In terms of IC, the overall goal of stretching is to relax the pelvic floor—but the pelvic floor is a complex network of muscles. It's not as simple as stretching a single muscle, such as a hamstring or quad. Fortunately, there are ways to target the pelvic floor directly, and these are the most important stretches you can do. So, if your time is limited on a certain day and you can't complete your full stretching routine, these are the ones to focus on.

The position of squatting naturally relaxes the pelvic floor. It's one of the reasons so many cultures around the world independently developed a tradition of squatting while urinating or defecating. Through much of human history, women even gave birth to children while squatting to take advantage of the relaxed position of the pelvic floor. The entire pelvic floor is able to release when you're in a squatting position. You may not feel it in the same way as you feel a muscle stretching, but the nature of this position forces the pelvic floor to open.

Pelvic Floor Squat Stretch

The best way to get the pelvic floor to relax is with a deep squat. Start with your feet shoulder-width apart and your toes pointed slightly outward. If you're new to this position, place your back against a wall for support. Keep your back straight, bend your knees, and squat down until your rear end is about six inches from the ground. This is a very deep squat—your hamstrings should be touching your calves. Don't stop the stretch halfway down, as your pelvic floor won't benefit if you don't get to the final position. Make sure to keep your heels on the floor and don't rise up on your toes. You'll feel an urge to tilt backward, which is why the wall can come in handy. When you're down in the final squatting position, place your elbows inside your thighs and work to spread your legs wider, increasing the stretch of the pelvic floor and inner thighs.

Once in the full squatting position, relax there and breathe deeply for a moment. Imagine your sit bones spreading apart. To get the full benefit of the stretch, consciously relax the pelvic floor by imagining you're about to start urinating: Some people describe this as feeling like the pelvic floor is dropping. The sense of release and relaxation should be the same that you feel when you first start to pee.

This can be a physically demanding stretch, especially if you have any problems with your hips or knees. If that's true for you, you can do a very similar stretch while lying on your back. However, if you *are* able to do it, know that it does have significant benefits over the supine version, with gravity working on your side and a more functional motion to relax the pelvic floor.

Happy Baby

This is essentially the same position as the pelvic floor squat stretches, but you're lying on your back instead of standing. Use a firm surface, such as a carpeted floor or yoga mat. Start by lying on your back with your knees up, feet flat on the floor. Now, bring both of your knees up toward your chest and grasp your legs at your knees, ankles, or the instep of your foot, depending on your flexibility level. Your feet should be close together and your knees flared wide, making a V with your legs. When you're at the end position, hold it, breathe deeply, and mentally recreate that moment when you first start to urinate. You should feel your pelvic floor dropping.

Support your head and upper shoulders with a pillow, if necessary. Your abdominal muscles should be relaxed during this stretch: You're not doing ab crunches. Hold the position for at least one minute. When you release the position, notice how different your pelvic floor feels. You may even notice an immediate change or easing in your pain and symptoms during these stretches.

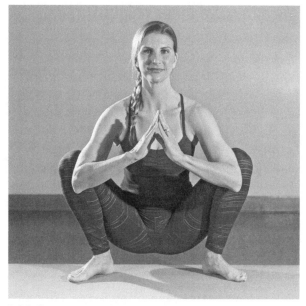

Pelvic floor squat stretch

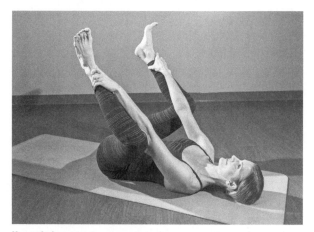

Happy baby

Relaxing the Inner Thighs

The close relationship between the bladder and the inner thighs means this is an important muscle group to stretch and relax. The bladder typically refers pain to this area, so most IC patients have tenderness and tightness in the muscles of the inner thighs. By working on these muscles you can alleviate pain in the bladder region, as well. These muscles are also important because, like almost all muscles in the region, they attach to the pelvis. Any tightness in the inner thighs exerts force on the pelvis and can lead to dysfunction and increased IC symptoms.

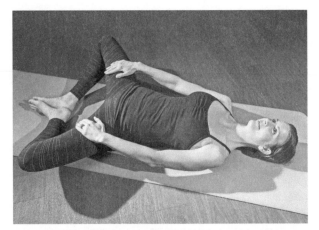

There are two types of inner thigh muscles:

1. Adductors: long muscles that go all the way from the pubic bone to the knee, running the entire length of the thigh

2. Groin muscles: short muscles that run from the pubic bone to the mid-thigh

We need to address both sets of muscles with a stretching program.

Butterfly Stretch

Start this stretch by lying on your back with your knees raised and pointed to the ceiling, and your feet flat on the floor. Let your knees slowly open and fall outward. You should feel a stretch in your upper inner thigh. If you have limited flexibility or are doing this stretch for the first time, the inner thighs may try to tighten to prevent the legs from falling further open. If you feel your inner thighs tightening or if there's any pain in your outside hip, slide a pillow underneath your outer thigh to support the weight of your legs and allow the inner thigh to relax more completely. As always, continue to work on deep breathing and relaxation during this stretch.

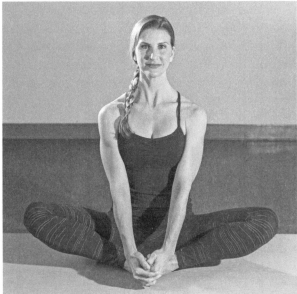

Butterfly stretch

If your inner thighs are too tight to perform this stretch comfortably, you can work on one leg at a time. Start in the same position, but only allow one leg to fall to the outside while keeping the sole of the other foot on the floor. This is less effective at stretching the inner thighs than the double-leg version, so graduate to the full stretch when you are able.

This stretch can also be done sitting up, with the soles of your feet pressed together. Your arms can rest on your legs to deepen the stretch. This can be a great position while doing something else at the same time, such as watching television or reading, but it makes deep breathing a little more challenging. For this reason, the supine version is preferred for the best and most relaxing stretch, but both are effective.

Chair Stretch

This stretch is a combination stretch that works on both the long muscles of the inner thighs and the hamstrings. Find a convenient chair or surface, such as a table, dresser, or kitchen counter. (The height of the surface isn't important.) Start with your feet wider than shoulder width apart, toes pointing slightly outward, about two feet away from the surface. Keeping your knees and back straight, fold your body over toward the surface and rest your elbows on top. If you're feeling a stretch already, you can hold the position here.

To get a deeper stretch, keep your feet planted and push your rear end away from the surface. You should be feeling a stretch along the backs of your legs in your hamstrings. While holding this stretch, imagine someone pulling your tailbone toward the ceiling and dropping your stomach toward the ground. This is the hamstring portion of the stretch, so hold it here for at least one minute.

Without moving your feet or arms, slightly bend one knee while keeping the pelvis back. Resist the urge to pitch forward. Leaning slightly in the direction of your bent leg, you should very quickly feel a stretch running down the inner thigh of your straight leg. Hold this for at least one minute, and then switch to the other side. This stretches the inner thigh and groin muscles and can help decrease bladder symptoms.

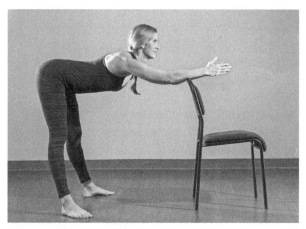

Chair stretch

Relaxing the Front of the Thighs

When you have bladder pain, all the muscles in the front of the thighs can tense up. The two important muscles here are the quads and the hip flexors. The quads are the big muscles on the front of your thigh. They allow you to kick and to swing the feet forward as you walk. Your hip flexors attach to the spine and run through the pelvic floor to the thigh, and are responsible for lifting your leg as you march in place. Sitting, driving, lying in the fetal position—essentially, doing any of the things humans do—tend to shorten these hip flexors. There are several stretches that target the quads, but the hip flexors are even more important to the proper functioning of the pelvic floor. They're where you should focus your stretching.

Mini-Lunge (Hip Flexor) Stretch

With your feet together, take a step forward, about 50 percent longer than your normal stride. Both feet should be flat on the floor and facing forward. To help with balance, do this stretch near a wall or table. Fighting the natural tendency of the body to twist, align your pelvis as much as possible with your front leg so your torso is aimed directly over your leading foot: You may already feel the stretch in your back leg in this position. If you're able, gradually bend your front knee and enhance the stretch, which you should feel in your upper inner thigh, right near your groin. Hold this stretch for at least one minute, and then switch legs.

This stretch has multiple benefits for IC patients. In addition to stretching the hip flexors, it also works on the calves. The nerves in your calf run all the way up your leg and through the pelvic floor, so releasing tension in the calf is beneficial. To focus on the calf portion of the stretch, you can increase the length of the lunge forward while trying to keep your back heel on the floor. You may have seen runners doing this stretch by pushing up against a wall or another solid object.

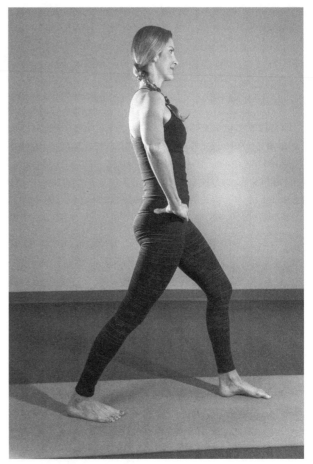

Mini-lunge (hip flexor) stretch

Relaxing the Abdomen

Your abdominal muscles attach directly over your bladder, so tightness in those muscles can put pressure on the organ. And when they're very tight, they can actually inhibit your bladder's ability to fill completely. Although we're conditioned to tighten and strengthen these ab muscles in pursuit of a six-pack, let's face it—that ship has sailed for most of us. Anyway, stretching muscles doesn't make them smaller or less prominent: It just prevents them from causing harm as they constantly tug on the surrounding tissue. There can also be a lot of residual inflammation trapped in the abdominal region from the bladder and pelvic floor dysfunction of interstitial cystitis.

Cobra Stretch

Lie face down on the floor and place your hands on either side of your chest, as if you were going to do a pushup. Point your toes so the tops of your feet contact the floor. Slowly, imagining you're stretching one vertebra at a time, extend your arms to lift your head and neck. Keep your pelvis glued to the ground as you lift yourself up with your arms and breathe deeply. You should feel a pull in your abdominal muscles. If you have back pain with this stretch or are unable to extend your arms, you can just come up onto your elbows. This will lift the torso more gently and will stretch the abdominal muscles. Hold this stretch for at least one minute, concentrating on long, deep breaths.

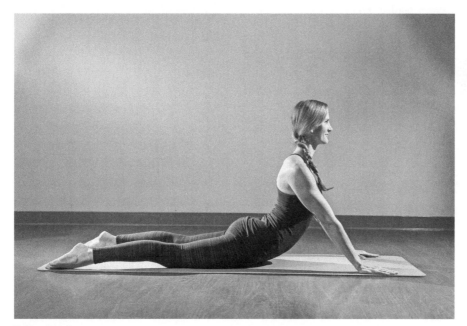

Cobra stretch

Relaxing the Gluteal Muscles

The gluteal muscles, or glutes, are the muscles that cushion your buttocks. The nerves that supply the bladder pass through the glute muscles, so this is an area in which tightness tends to build up and irritate the already-sensitive nerves.

Figure 4 Stretch

Start on your back with your feet flat on the floor and knees bent. Place your right ankle on the front of your left knee. This creates a keyhole, or the open part of the number 4. You may feel the stretch already in your right glute muscles, stretching from your sit bone toward the outside of your hip. If you are able, reach both hands forward. Clasp them behind your left knee and gently pull it back toward you, which should enhance the stretch. When you are finished, switch legs and stretch the other side.

If you're unable to tolerate this stretch, or if your muscles are so tight you can't get your ankle to your knee, you can modify the exercise. From the same starting position, simply reach forward and pull your knee straight back to your chest. This doesn't reach quite the same range of muscles as the original stretch, so if you become able to do the Figure 4 stretch, you should do so. This stretch also relieves tension in the lower back, which can affect IC patients.

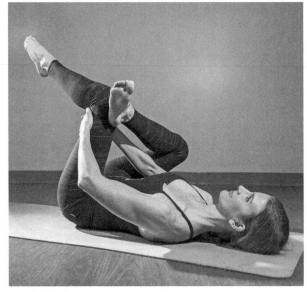

Figure 4 stretch

Take Time for Yourself

The benefits of self-care are directly proportional to the amount of time you're able to invest in it. Completing one full rotation through these stretches takes only about ten minutes.

I recommend that my patients do these stretches at least twice a day, but the more you do them, the faster you can improve. Many patients get creative about incorporating them into their daily lives. Instead of just sitting on the couch to watch your favorite TV show, you can also do the butterfly, figure 4, and abdominal stretching. Opening mail? Lean over the counter as you read it to stretch your hamstrings and inner thighs. Calling your mother? That's a great time to do a mini-lunge to stretch your groin. The more tension and stress you can release from these muscles, the better.

Stretch	**Time**
Pelvic floor squat stretch or happy baby	1 minute
Butterfly inner thigh stretch	1 minute
Chair hamstring and inner thigh stretch	3 minutes
Mini-lunge inner thigh stretch	2 minutes
Cobra abdominal stretch	1 minute
Figure 4 stretch	2 minutes
Total	*10 minutes*

Skin Rolling and Fascial Release

Fascia is the connective tissue that lies between the muscles and the skin. If you've cooked a raw chicken, you've probably seen it—the white fibrous tissue that slides over the chicken breast that you often cut or pull off. Researchers are finding out that this connective tissue plays a far larger role in our lives than we previously thought.

Connective tissue is made up of two parts: collagen fibers and a fluid extra-cellular matrix. When you have chronic pelvic pain and dysfunction, as with interstitial cystitis, your body responds by rushing the healing molecules and emergency responders to the area. But the influx of inflammation is greater than your body's ability to clear it out.

The fluid of your connective tissue, which started out thin and slippery like olive oil, turns to a runny oatmeal consistency from the excess inflammation trapped in it. When this happens, the connective tissue stops acting as a lubricated surface between your skin and muscles. The skin begins to adhere to the muscles underneath and contributes to the tightness and pain in the area. Medical research, or your physical therapist, may refer to this condition as panniculosis. With IC, this frequently occurs over the bladder and inner thighs. Blood vessels run through the fascia, so dysfunction there can reduce blood flow to the area. Fascial dysfunction can inhibit muscle function, bladder filling, and pelvic floor relaxation, and can create painful trigger points in the fascia itself that contribute to the cycle of pelvic pain.

Fascial release and skin rolling aim to counteract this problem. Physical therapy will always work to address the fascial component, but there are three ways to work on the fascia yourself. Short videos demonstrating these techniques are available at PelvicSanity.com.

Fascial Elongation

Fascial elongation is the gentlest form of fascial release, and is a good starting place if you're new to treatment or are extremely tender to the touch. In this method, you place the palm of both hands on an area of concern; the abdominal muscles are the best place to start. The anchor hand gently presses and holds on the skin, while the glide hand slowly slides across the skin away from it. You can use a bit of lotion to reduce friction. Vary the direction and angle at which you pull away from the anchor hand. You may feel a slight burning sensation on your skin, almost like a rug burn, if the fascia is sensitive. That burning isn't coming from the friction on the skin, but from the fascia underneath.

With the anchor hand in place on the stomach, just above the belly button, allow the glide hand to move away down your abdomen. These strokes can be short, finishing at the pubic bone, but you'll also want to do longer strokes that run all the way to the inner thigh. Once you have completed these strokes in all directions, move the anchor hand to the inner thigh, and repeat the process on both legs. Spend two or three minutes in each spot before moving on to the next. Afterward, you may feel a rush of blood to the area, or see the skin turn red. Both are indications that blood flow is returning to the area to clear out the inflammation and dysfunction.

Fascial Distraction (Clock Method)

Fascial distraction (clock method) is a technique that clears up adhesions in the fascia between the skin and muscle underneath. Lying on your back, grip about an inch (centimeter) of skin on your abdomen between your fingers and pull up, away from the body. If you haven't done fascial release before, or if this area is extremely tender, this may be uncomfortable. Pull the skin up and feel the stretch of the fascia releasing.

When you're able to, hold and pull the skin along the face of an imaginary clock. Stretch it toward you (twelve o'clock) and away (six o'clock). When you're doing this, note which direction is more restricted or uncomfortable. Gently pull the skin, first in the direction that's easier, until it relaxes, and then in the direction of greater restriction.

Once both directions feel less tender, change your angle so you're moving between one and seven o'clock, then two and eight o'clock, and so on until the area is free of restriction. Then find another area on your abdomen and repeat the process. You should do this throughout every area of your abdomen (at least four sites), and then on your inner thighs.

Skin Rolling

Skin rolling starts the same way as the fascial distraction method, by pulling up an inch or so of skin from your body—but instead of holding it there, you'll roll your fingers over the skin. Keeping your thumbs locked, slowly roll your fingers down, and slide your thumbs behind them.

This may be uncomfortable and may feel like there are Rice Krispies underneath your skin, cracking and popping as you loosen the fascia. Other patients describe it as "gunky"—you're actually feeling the inflammation trapped beneath the surface. Especially early on, be gentle with yourself in this technique. Some areas may still be too tender for this. In that case, use the fascial distraction method on that problem area until your fingers can glide over it.

■ Abdominal Scars

If you've had surgery or injury to your abdominal area, scars may have become stuck to the tissue underneath. This condition can make skin rolling more difficult and painful—but even more necessary.

A C-section is one of the most common scars that pose problems for IC patients. The incision is made right over the bladder and reaches all the way into the uterus. And, if it wasn't maintained properly during healing, it can be stuck to the tissue underneath, affecting your bladder. Other surgeries that can affect this abdominal and pelvic area include appendectomies, hysterectomies, laparoscopic surgeries, prostate removals, gall bladder removal, cosmetic surgeries, such as tummy tucks, and any other pelvic surgery. Be especially mindful of any surgery with a belly button incision. Even if the surgeries are "minimally invasive," there are still incisions that can scar and adhere.

The same fascial release techniques can be used on any of these scars, but they may also need additional attention. In an ideal world, a scar—no matter how old—should move just as freely as the connective tissue around it. However, patients often aren't informed that they should work on freeing the scar as soon as it heals to make sure it doesn't adhere to surrounding tissue. If you're doing self-work on an incision after a procedure, wait six weeks after surgery to make sure it has fully healed, or until you have permission from your physical therapist or surgeon.

To work on the scarred area, use the same fascial release techniques directly on the scar. By picking the skin up and rolling it, you break some of the connections the scar has made, allowing the skin to move freely again and restoring proper function to the area. A physical therapist can be of great assistance here, particular if the scar is strongly stuck or painful.

Trigger Point Release

After you have worked to clear up the problems in the fascia, you can address the knots in the muscles underneath. Clearing the fascia first has several advantages when it comes to trigger point release. First, it should be substantially less uncomfortable than it would be otherwise, because you won't be pressing down on dysfunctional fascia on top of a muscle knot. Plus, there will be more blood flow to the area, which will help the muscles respond to your self-massage. Finally, clearing the fascia can also help release the muscular trigger points, making them even easier to eliminate.

External Trigger Point Release

For this trigger point release, use a little bit of lotion on your fingertips so your hands glide over the skin. With gentle pressure, you should be able to feel the position of a knot underneath the surface of the muscle. When you reach this spot, let your fingers linger there, and apply consistent pressure to it for ninety seconds. You should feel some discomfort during this process; you may feel a burning sensation or even pain that's referred to another part of the body. It's always surprising the first time you put pressure on your inner thighs and realize it's reproducing your bladder pain or urgency—but that's exactly why these self-care techniques are so important.

As you hold the pressure for ninety seconds, you should feel a bit of a change in the sensation. If the muscle is ready, you may feel the knot dissolve underneath your fingertips. If the trigger point doesn't release completely, that's okay. Simply glide your fingers down to the next tender or knotted spot and repeat the process. Sometimes you'll come back to the original trigger point after you've done some additional self-massage or fascial release, and find that it breaks up easily. All trigger points and tightness in the muscles are related; by working on one, you can make the others easier to address.

You should perform this trigger point release in the same areas surrounding the pelvis you've been working on for fascial release: inner thighs, outer thighs, the length of your quad muscles down to your knee, and on your gluteal muscles over your buttocks and hips. (The only area where it's harder to release trigger points is the abdomen; stick with fascial release there.) Once you finish working an area, stretch it immediately using your stretching routine. It's like untangling a set of knotted headphones: After you release the knot, the muscle may have a tendency to curl back into place; prevent that by stretching the muscle.

You should notice a change in how it feels to stretch. Maybe you get more length on your stretch, or feel your place of restriction move. These trigger points are often what you're feeling when you hit the end range of a stretch and feel like your body can't go any further. When you release them, you'll be surprised by how different stretching feels.

It may be beneficial to have someone else help you with external trigger point release. If you have a supportive and willing partner, he or she can learn these techniques, as well. You may also consider a local massage therapist who will already be familiar with trigger point release—it's the basis for most therapeutic massages.

■ External Trigger Point Release Tools

Now that you know how to release trigger points with your hands and fingers, there are a few other tools that might be useful. A foam roller is a cylindrical piece of foam that can help you put pressure on the trigger points of your legs and glutes. You'll approach it in the same way that you work with your hands. Lying on the floor with a leg over the foam roller, slide your leg over the roller until you find an uncomfortable trigger point. Once you reach the knot, use your body weight to apply steady pressure to the point for the same ninety seconds.

You can also gently rock against the foam roller to help dissolve the knot. Ease the pressure by changing how much of your body weight you support on your hands and opposite leg, and how much you put on the roller. If you have significant tenderness from your trigger points, this may be a bit intense for you the first few times. In that case, return to working with your hands and progress to the foam roller once you've cleared the fascial tension and worked on the trigger points manually.

Once you get comfortable with it, the foam roller can make trigger point release faster and save your hands from the work of self-massage. You can work over your inner thighs, quads, outer thighs, and gluteal muscles with the foam roller, moving from your knee all the way up to your groin or hips. As with all forms of trigger point release, make sure to stretch afterward. You can find foam rollers in many sporting goods stores or online. You might look for one that's a little softer—or with more "give"—than those geared toward athletes, because your trigger points are more likely to be painful and sensitive.

You can also use a tennis ball in place of the foam roller to give you a little more control over the spot that you're releasing, particularly on your gluteal muscles. Or, use a smaller plastic self-rolling massager or "stick": You grasp the handles and run it over your skin, just like a foam roller. This has the advantage of being smaller and more portable than a full foam roller, and it gives you a bit more control over the pressure you exert.

Internal Trigger Point Release

The same trigger point release methods we just described can be used internally, directly on the pelvic floor. While this may be unfamiliar at first, patients soon become experts at self-care and realize it's no different than working on an area externally. These internal trigger points need to be cleared before your daily symptoms can be eliminated. This can be done in physical therapy, as well, but self-care allows you to do your own maintenance to solidify the gains of PT.

Women have the choice between intravaginal and intra-rectal trigger point release: The same internal muscles can be reached and cleared of knots and trigger points regardless of the entry point. Typically, female IC patients start vaginally because of the close proximity to the bladder and urethra and the muscles that control them.

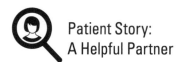

Patient Story:
A Helpful Partner

Partners of IC patients can feel frustrated and helpless. In my practice, I often invite the partners of patients into a portion of a treatment session so they can learn about the pelvic floor and how to help. One patient brought her husband, Gregg, to one of our sessions.

At first, Gregg was embarrassed and reluctant to be in the room while his wife was receiving treatment. He had difficulty even concentrating on learning basic information about the condition. We started by teaching him external fascial and trigger point release skills, so he could help his wife with self-massage on her inner thighs, abdomen, and glutes.

But about a month after our initial visit, Gregg realized how much he was helping his wife, and he asked about internal techniques, as well. He learned about internal trigger point release, and was amazed that he could actually feel the source of his wife's symptoms. Afterward, the couple felt they could tackle a symptom flare together, and Gregg had a much better understanding of his wife's condition—and, more importantly, a way to help her.

■ *Vaginal Trigger Point Release*

Imagine your vagina as a clock (guys, you may be tempted to skip this section, but many of these same techniques are used rectally for men). The top of the clock, twelve o'clock, is closest to you and your pubic bone, with the bottom at six o'clock at your perineum. This orientation will soon become very familiar, helping you navigate your pelvic floor. Lie back in a comfortable position with your knees bent. Using a small amount of personal lubricant, slowly insert a finger just inside the vagina, only to the first knuckle. Now, you'll perform the same type of trigger point release that you have already been doing externally. Start at the two o'clock position (on your right), and gently press

and hold for ninety seconds. Then move to three o'clock and on through the rest of the positions until you reach ten o'clock, holding at each trigger point you find for ninety seconds. *Don't press between ten and two o'clock, right beneath your pubic bone: That's your bladder and urethra.*

As you move through the positions, make a mental note of what you find. Some spots can be tight and painful in the immediate location only, while other trigger points will reproduce your symptoms. Some will refer pain to a different site in the pelvic floor or surrounding region. Other spots may be completely healthy, and already free of sensitive knots. Releasing all trigger points will be important for symptom relief.

FEMALE PELVIC FLOOR ANATOMY

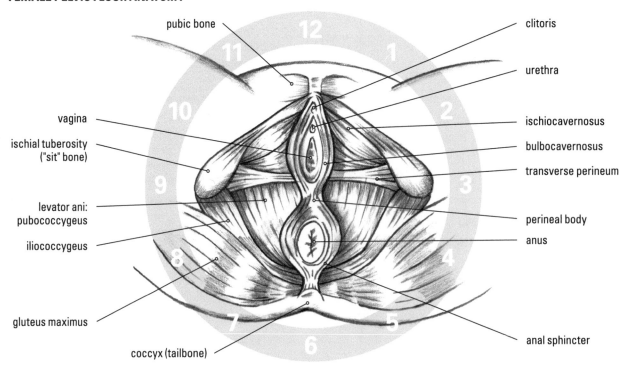

With IC, many patients have a lot of tightness in the upper areas of the clock, between two and three o'clock and nine and ten o'clock. These muscles are closest to the bladder and urethra, the ones that control the flow of urine. When they have been overtaxed by the urinary frequency of interstitial cystitis, they can become knotted and painful. At the bottom of the clock, you may reproduce feelings you have with painful sex; this is the area most often responsible for problems with intercourse. As you get more familiar with your pelvic floor, you'll know where to anticipate trigger points and where your personal problem spots are. And this part of the process doesn't take long: You can make a full circuit through the areas of the pelvic floor in about ten to fifteen minutes.

Once you've made a full rotation through the pelvic floor at this depth, it's time to go a little bit deeper. Slide the finger in another half-inch (1 cm) or so, up to the second joint in your finger, and repeat the internal massage. You may notice problems in the same "hour," or in different areas. Continue to press and hold for ninety seconds in each spot, avoiding the areas right underneath your pubic bone. Once you've completed this rotation, go slightly deeper, up to the third knuckle on your finger, and repeat it at this depth. Never go deeper than two or three inches (5 to 7.5 cm) when doing internal work as you may encounter more sensitive areas and nerve endings. A trained PT might work on deeper trigger points, and may even instruct you on how to reach them yourself—but don't try to reach them without specific instructions from your pelvic floor physical therapist. A full internal trigger point release session should take about twenty to thirty minutes. As you improve, you'll become aware of your specific problem areas, and will be able to shorten the process using a more targeted approach.

After you have identified and relieved the pelvic floor of trigger points—hopefully with the help of a physical therapist—you'll eventually perform internal self-massage just for maintenance:

It ensures that no problems are brewing under the surface. Remember that these trigger points can develop without immediately causing symptoms, so making sure your pelvic floor stays healthy is vital in sustaining your improvements. Even patients who have eliminated their symptoms should still spend about five minutes twice a week clearing their pelvic floor trigger points to ensure they don't return.

■ *Rectal Trigger Point Release*

Men release internal trigger points within the rectum, and women may also use this method on the advice of their physical therapists. Rectal trigger point release works in a very similar way to intravaginal release. Lying flat on your back with your knees bent, again imagine the face of a clock. The top of the clock, twelve o'clock, is facing the pubic bone and genitalia, while the six o'clock is on the bottom near the tailbone. Using a personal lubricant, place gentle pressure against the anus for thirty seconds until it relaxes. When you are able, insert a finger up to about the first knuckle, approximately ½ inch (1 cm) inside. Starting at one o'clock—just barely inside the anus—apply gentle pressure and feel for a trigger point. When you find one, hold the pressure there for ninety seconds and then move on to the next position at two o'clock. Work your way clockwise from one o'clock to five o'clock. Skip the very bottom of the clock: This is your tailbone. *You won't harm yourself if you do touch your tailbone, but massaging bone is rarely helpful. Your physical therapist can actually fix a poorly aligned tailbone, which may be causing pain, but you should leave this area alone.*

Start again at seven o'clock and work your way back up the other side. *Men: Don't feel for trigger points between eleven and one o'clock because this is the prostate area.* Again, make a note of what you find. Do any of the trigger points reproduce your urinary symptoms or IC pain? If so, focus on improving those areas, as they'll result in direct improvements in your symptoms. As with intravaginal release, trigger points on the top of the clock (between nine and three o'clock) tend to reproduce urinary urgency, urethral burning, and bladder pain. Trigger points in the lower half of the clock are more likely to cause low back pain, hip pain, tailbone pain, or pain with sex. Once you get to know your pelvic floor, you can often go straight to the trigger point that's causing your symptoms and release it for immediate relief.

As with intravaginal release, now it's time to move slightly deeper. Slide your finger in up to the next joint and repeat the exercise. Once you have completed another revolution around the clock, you can go a little bit deeper—up to the knuckle—for the final circuit around the clock. Again, don't go any deeper on your own unless instructed by your physical therapist.

■ *Internal Trigger Point Release Tools*
Once you are comfortable manually identifying and releasing internal trigger points, you may find a crystal wand, such as TheraWand, to be helpful. This is an S-shaped tool about the size of your hand that can be used in place of your finger to find and treat internal pelvic floor trigger points. You use it to go through the different hours of the clock, just like you would with your fingers. Patients often find it easier to reach their trigger points with the crystal wand, and most patients use it for the maintenance stage once they become proficient in internal self-care. There are different versions of this tool for the vagina and rectum. They're difficult to find in stores; look online, or your pelvic floor physical therapist may have one for sale.

This can be a useful tool, especially when you're doing a lot of self-work. However, the crystal wand doesn't have as much give as your finger, so make sure you're comfortable doing the internal massage manually before progressing to the less-forgiving tool. Remember, you should never enter deeper than about two inches (5 cm), in either the vagina or rectum.

For women with pelvic floor dysfunction or sexual pain, even inserting a finger into the vagina can be painful. In these cases, a dilator may be an important tool for your self-care. The dilator is designed to gently stretch the vaginal wall and tissue of the vagina. This can release some of the tightness and allow you to work on specific trigger points within the vagina. These dilators often come in sets of four, gradually increasing in size. As your pelvic floor begins to release, you can begin increasing the size of the dilator. This can also be a helpful way for women who have pain with sex to reduce symptoms and become more comfortable with penetration.

Bladder Training with Interstitial Cystitis

Your physical therapist or doctor may recommend bladder training, where you work actively to retrain your bladder to increase time between voiding. This is a common treatment technique with overactive bladder or incontinence, and has been shown to reduce frequency in some interstitial cystitis patients. The first step is keeping a voiding diary (see chapter 4), detailing how often you use the bathroom. Then set a deliberate schedule where you try to use the bathroom at a specific time, regardless of whether or not you feel an urge at that point. For instance, if you were typically urinating every fifty minutes, you might start by scheduling urinations on the hour, and working to hold it in until you reach the specified time. Over time, the intervals between these bathroom breaks increase, and can make your bladder more comfortable with holding in urine for longer.

This treatment method isn't appropriate for every patient, though. Patients with pelvic floor dysfunction already have tight muscles; further clenching them to hold in urine can cause pain and exacerbate pelvic floor tightness. Talk to your physical therapist before beginning bladder training.

WEEKLY TRACKING CHART

	Mon	Tues	Wed	Thur	Fri	Sat	Sun	Total
Stretching routine (#1)								
Stretching routine (#2)								
Fascial release								
External trigger point release								
Internal trigger point release								

Looking for a way to make your self-care routine a healthy habit? A weekly chart, such as this one, can remind you of your daily routine and record how well you're doing with your regimen. Place a similar chart on your refrigerator (a printable version is available at PelvicSanity.com), and add a checkmark in each box when you complete your daily routine. Tally the week's totals to see how you've done. Ideally, your goal is to complete your stretching routine twice daily, and to add at least one other self-care activity (fascial release, external, or internal trigger point release) each day.

Takeaways

- **"Self-care" doesn't mean "alone."** Although the title of this chapter is self-care, you don't have to do all of this by yourself. A significant other can be taught to do these techniques and can help you with them, or you can ask a massage therapist to focus on the trigger points of your thigh, gluteal, and lower back muscles.

- **Self-care is a critical part of your IC journey.** By combining stretching with fascia and trigger point release, you address some of the underlying problems created by interstitial cystitis. These self-care treatments allow you to take control of your condition. This part of your treatment is entirely up to you; make the most of it.

FOOD AS MEDICINE:

The Role of Diet in IC

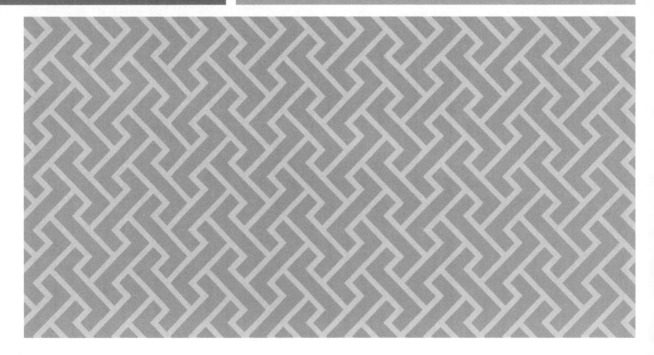

Diet is an extremely important—but often misunderstood—part of the interstitial cystitis journey. Surveys show that somewhere between 80 and 96 percent of IC patients have food sensitivities that trigger symptoms. Eliminating certain foods and beverages from your diet can significantly reduce pain and urinary urgency. Ultimately, your diet is unique to you, and depends on how you respond to different foods.

There are a few common trigger foods. These include citrus fruits and juices, caffeine, alcohol, carbonated beverages, artificial sweeteners, tomatoes, and spicy foods. While these are the most likely triggers, you may be sensitive to all, some, or none. A disciplined approach will let you learn what you can and can't eat, and your symptom diary can be an important tool in determining which foods or drinks tend to cause symptoms to flare.

Myths abound regarding what you can and can't eat. This chapter examines the truth behind these misconceptions, and gives you the facts on how small changes to your diet can have a big impact on your IC symptoms.

There Is No Formal "IC Diet"

Food sensitivities are different for everyone. And there's no such thing as a formal "IC diet" to govern everything you eat and drink. In fact, one study found no difference between strict adherence to a highly restrictive "IC diet" and an individualized approach to identifying and eliminating only your personal trigger foods. In a large 2011 study, conducted by a partnership between researchers from the University of South Florida and the Interstitial Cystitis Association, IC patients were asked about 344 different foods. The authors showed the vast majority of foods had no negative impact at all for most patients. Another study from Long Island University found that just thirty-five specific items tended to flare symptoms, and that most people are only sensitive to a fraction of them.

Myth Alert! Patients Need to Follow a Specific "IC Diet" to Get Better

Fact: Everyone is different. You need to identify your unique trigger foods and drinks and eliminate them from your diet.

The origin of the "IC diet" myth may have been a comprehensive IC food list circulated by the Interstitial Cystitis Association (ICA), an important patient advocacy group that has been crucial in raising awareness and research funds for interstitial cystitis. Responding to patient requests for a diet list, they put out an exhaustive list of foods anecdotally reported to be triggers for some patients.

Though meant as a helpful patient resource, seeing all the reported trigger foods listed like that can be overwhelming. The ICA acknowledges that this food list is not reflective of the majority of IC patients—but, unfortunately, some people have interpreted that resource as an authoritative "IC diet," which simply doesn't exist.

While at least one person may have reported a sensitivity to a food or beverage on that list, no one has reported a sensitivity to *all* of them. In fact, in a survey of more than 2,000 patients, the ICA found that simply eliminating your trigger foods was just as effective as trying to follow the entire list of possible dietary restrictions—and much easier!

Patient Story:
A Damaging Diet

Sammy had been diagnosed with IC, plus fibromyalgia and irritable bowel syndrome. After seeing an online "IC diet" on an Internet forum, she became convinced that her diet was responsible for her symptoms. So, she embarked on a gluten-free, soy-free, dairy-free, inflammation-free, sugar-free diet. I couldn't help but wonder what she actually *was* eating.

Well, she'd been so scared of the foods' effect on her symptoms that she'd basically limited herself to chicken and rice—for breakfast, lunch, and dinner—because she'd read that those were the safest foods for IC. Her hair was thin, her nails were brittle, and her complexion had a yellow-gray tinge. When she entered my clinic, Sammy was clinically malnourished. I referred her to a nutritionist who specializes in pain conditions, such as interstitial cystitis, to help her find a balanced diet that would accommodate her food limitations.

Patients are often frightened by what they read online, and eliminate things from their diets without adding anything to compensate. But it's just as important to get a healthy variety of foods, nutrients, and nourishment as it is to eliminate trigger foods. So, don't just avoid negative triggers: Actively work toward a healthier diet, which will benefit your overall well-being.

Researchers still don't have an explanation for why certain foods are symptom triggers, or why they differ so much between patients. Some people don't seem to have food triggers at all. There doesn't seem to be an underlying connection between the most common food triggers. So you'll need to identify your own personal food sensitivities.

Acidic Foods, Acidic Urine, and pH

One persistent myth is that food sensitivity is due to the acid content of your urine. This seems logical at first. If the bladder lining is compromised or permeable, urine may penetrate and come into contact with the sensitive nerves of the exposed bladder underneath; the more acidic the urine, the more it has the potential to burn and cause symptoms. Researchers from the University of British Columbia set out to prove this theory in 2005. They catheterized brave IC volunteers and actually put (their own) urine back into their bladders. Some patients got naturally acidic urine, while the control group had the acid neutralized so the urine inserted was neutral instead. The researchers expected the acidic urine to be much more painful. But instead, they were surprised to find no difference between the two groups—the urine's acidity didn't seem to matter at all.

The other aspect of this myth that can confuse patients is the idea that acidic foods should be avoided because they end up making the urine more acidic. This theory is used to explain why some foods containing citric acid, such as citrus fruits and juices, are common trigger foods. However, it's not nearly as simple as "acid in, acid out." The truth is there's an incredibly complex relationship between what you eat, your blood chemistry, and what ends up leaving your bladder. And if your food's acidity were to blame for IC symptoms, a simple antacid would have a far greater effect in reducing acid levels than avoiding acidic foods completely.

Chemistry Review: pH

The measurement of how acidic or basic a substance is, on a scale of 0 to 14, is called pH. Water is considered perfectly neutral, at a pH of 7. Any pH level *below 7* is considered *acidic*, while anything *over 7* is considered *basic* or *alkaline*. On one end of the spectrum are strong acids, such as sulfuric acid, that can melt and burn what they touch. On the other end are strong bases, such as ammonia, lye, and bleach, which can also cause burns to the skin.

The pH of a food or drink at the moment of consumption has almost no relationship to what it does inside your body. Many alkaline substances are metabolized into acids within the body, while acidic foods can become basic when they're processed inside you. A great example is the lemon—one of the most acidic edible foods. The pH of lemon juice is approximately 2, since it's composed of almost 5 percent citric acid. But, after they're eaten, lemons actually turn highly basic inside the body. In fact, researchers found that drinking lemon juice actually raised the pH of the urine!

Levels of pH are most important when it comes to your bloodstream. There's a very narrow range of blood pH that allows the body to function: Step outside this range and you'll find yourself in a coma, fighting for your life. That's why your body has become extremely efficient at making sure the acidity of your blood stays constant, and the kidneys and the urine they produce play a major role in regulating blood acidity. Your urine's pH can (naturally and greatly) fluctuate throughout the day, from a highly acidic pH of 4.5 up to a basic pH of 8. If the acidity of your urine were a primary factor in bladder symptoms, your pain would have wild variations throughout the day as the pH of the urine rises and falls.

It's important to debunk this myth because many patients end up trying to slash all acidic foods from their diets. Not only is this nearly impossible, it also means that following your diet is a full-time job. Plus, cutting out too many foods can make it difficult to get all the important nutrients your body needs. Don't make your diet any more restrictive than it has to be.

The Elimination Diet

So if a strict "IC diet" isn't necessary, and acidic foods aren't really the culprits, what's going on? Research hasn't yet been able to answer that question conclusively. Some foods and drinks may cause problems for IC patients because they irritate the bladder in everyone. Caffeine and alcohol, two common IC triggers, are diuretics that prompt more trips to the bathroom for everyone who consumes them. Combine that bladder irritation with the underlying problems of IC, and it's not surprising they top the list of irritating substances. Caffeine has a stimulant effect on the nervous system—which is why it helps keep you awake and alert—but it may also amplify pain signals to your brain. Other problem foods may have similar, undiscovered reasons for flaring symptoms, or there may be a commonality between them that researchers have yet to discover.

Experts agree the best way to address symptoms associated with food is through the elimination diet. The elimination diet is a method for determining which items are contributing to your symptoms. The first step is to remove all the usual suspects from your diet for two to four weeks. Kicking your morning coffee habit, passing up wine with dinner, or avoiding your favorite Indian restaurant might be tough, but it's worth it: You'll learn a lot about your condition and your food sensitivities. A good symptom log, as discussed in chapter 2, helps by giving an accurate account of your symptoms.

Keep in mind, too, that your sensitivities may not seem logical. For instance, some patients report flares with blueberries, but are fine eating raspberries. Or, you might be able to eat some citrus fruits without a problem, while others have instant consequences. Your sensitivities can also change over time. If you've gone without a treasured food or drink for a long time, it may be worth trying it again at some point to see whether your body's reaction to it has changed.

IC Trigger Foods

Several large surveys and research studies have identified the foods most commonly associated with symptoms in IC. They include:

- Alcoholic and carbonated beverages
- Artificial sweeteners
- Caffeine-containing drinks, such as coffee and tea
- Citrus fruits (lemons, limes, oranges, grapefruit, and tangerines)
- Cranberry juice
- Spicy foods
- Tomatoes

Remember, though, everyone is different. You may not have sensitivities to all, or any, items on this list. It is possible to have additional food sensitivities—but these are the primary culprits.

"When it comes to an IC-friendly diet, the bottom line is: Eat healthily and avoid your food triggers. That's it."

Specialty Diets

There's a lot of chatter about the benefits of specialty diets, each with strong advocates. You'll see recommendations for gluten-free, dairy-free, and Paleolithic diets, and other regimens. Some offer some specific benefits for IC patients, but much of what they propose is not necessary for improving symptoms of interstitial cystitis. When it comes to an IC-friendly diet, the bottom line is: Eat healthily and avoid your food triggers. That's it. Don't make it more complicated.

If you've been on a (healthy) specialty diet for a while and find it's working for you, great. You may want to make a few slight modifications to eliminate any other trigger foods you've found, but there's no reason to change things up. However, if you're just starting your journey with IC, you don't have to throw yourself into a hard-to-follow diet. We all have a finite amount of time, energy, and willpower, and you need to be smart about how you spend yours. You'll be much better off simply eliminating your food triggers and saving that extra energy for stretching, meditation, physical therapy, or something else that directly addresses the problem, rather than restricting yourself to a draconian diet.

Paleolithic Diet

The premise of the Paleolithic diet is to eat foods our ancestors ate before the advent of farming, approximately 10,000 years ago. This hunter-gatherer diet completely eliminates:

- Alcohol
- Coffee
- Dairy products (milk, cheese, butter)
- Grains (wheat, corn, rice)
- Legumes (beans and nuts)
- Processed foods
- Salt
- Sugar

By going Paleo, you automatically go dairy- and gluten-free. Instead, the diet encourages greater protein intake from meats and fish, and its carbohydrates come from fresh, nonstarchy fruits and vegetables.

While the Paleo diet has some important characteristics for IC patients, including eliminating some common IC triggers and an emphasis on fresh fruits and vegetables, it is one of the most restrictive diet types. If you're contemplating switching to the Paleo diet, you'll have to change your food-shopping and cooking habits completely. And this is an investment of time and energy that may not make the most sense for you if you've recently been diagnosed. But if you're already established in the Paleo diet, you can continue it with only slight modifications to avoid any additional trigger foods.

Dairy-Free Diet

A dairy-free diet works to reduce or eliminate lactose, a specific kind of sugar found in milk products, such as cheese, yogurt, and butter. This diet doesn't eliminate many common IC triggers, but, since many people with IC also experience irritable bowel syndrome, a dairy-free diet can be helpful if lactose irritates your IBS symptoms. Fortunately, there are very good replacement products available, including lactose-free milk, which is nearly indistinguishable from traditional milk. It can be made into lactose-free cheese, yogurt, and butter, so it shouldn't be too difficult to switch to a dairy-free diet if lactose is a problem for you.

Gluten-Free Diet

Based on the hypothesis that gluten sensitivity causes symptoms, such as intestinal discomfort, bloating, depression, anxiety, and a foggy mind, the gluten-free movement has been gaining momentum around the world. While some people are diagnosed with celiac disease or a wheat allergy, and certainly struggle when eating gluten, others don't have a specific diagnosis but still feel they have trouble processing it. There is a raging debate in the scientific and nutritional community over whether nonceliac gluten sensitivity exists. There is evidence—sometimes even from the same study—cited on both sides of the argument.

Practically speaking, going gluten-free can encourage you to avoid packaged and processed foods, and become more cognizant of your carbohydrate intake. While there is no conclusive evidence about gluten-free diets and IC, going gluten-free isn't harmful, and may have a positive benefit.

Dietary Supplements

Many people take supplements in conjunction with their particular diet or eating plan. In general, dietary supplements are not rigorously evaluated for their medical properties. The claims on bottles are not evaluated by any regulatory agency, so be cautious when relying on their marketing. That said, there are some supplements that have been reported in pilot studies, surveys, and anecdotally as helpful for IC. The best approach is, as always, to maximize the benefits of a treatment while minimizing side effects, and many of these supplements have a low incidence of negative effects. They may be an important addition to a holistic treatment plan.

Consulting a Nutritionist

For some patients, food sensitivity is the driving factor behind their IC symptoms. If you notice that you are highly sensitive to certain foods with your elimination diet, it may be worthwhile to consult a nutritionist. He or she can help you eliminate your trigger foods and replace them with healthy alternatives. There are fantastic nutritionists who specialize in designing diets for people with chronic pain conditions, such as IC. Even a few visits to get your diet on track can pay huge dividends in the longer term.

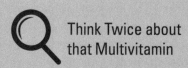

Think Twice about that Multivitamin

Lots of us take multivitamins without giving them much thought. After all, they can't do any harm and may do some good—right? As it turns out, that's not necessarily true for IC patients.

Vitamin C

We commonly reach for vitamin C when we're under the weather, and it's found in nearly all multivitamins. But researchers have found that vitamin C is often a food trigger for IC symptoms in its isolated form. (However, this isn't true for foods in which it occurs naturally: dozens of fruits and vegetables high in vitamin C almost never cause problems for patients.)

Vitamin B

In patient surveys, people with IC have also reported sensitivity to B-complex vitamins. Again, this effect seems to be isolated to the high-dosage, packaged form and doesn't seem to apply to foods naturally high in these important vitamins, which are important to energy levels and heart health. Foods high in B vitamins include leafy vegetables, fish, beans, and some grains and fruits.

You should be able to get your recommended daily amount of both vitamins by eating a healthy, balanced diet high in fruits and vegetables. Skip the pills and let your food be your medicine!

Calcium Glycerophosphate

A mineral supplement that generally works as an antacid, calcium glycerophosphate (Prelief) is one of the most studied supplements for interstitial cystitis treatment. In a large, uncontrolled trial of more than 200 patients, the supplement was shown to reduce both the pain and urgency of IC when taken immediately before trigger foods. Food sensitivities were reduced or eliminated in some patients. In a larger survey conducted by the Interstitial Cystitis Association, calcium glycerophosphate was the highest-rated supplement by the 2,000 responders, with nearly 75 percent reporting a positive effect. This is also one of the more popular supplements on the market for those with IC; in the survey, nearly half of the responders reported having tried calcium glycerophosphate.

How the supplement might reduce the symptoms of food triggers remains unclear. As you already learned, putting acidic foods into the body doesn't equate to acidic urine, and it's doubtful that calcium glycerophosphate or other antacids significantly influence the urine's pH. And, even if they did, studies have shown that the acidity of the urine probably has no effect on interstitial cystitis in the majority of patients. None of the studies that evaluate calcium glycerophosphate have been blinded, so the placebo effect may play a role in the reported benefits. However, it's clear that a substantial number of patients note a reduction in food-triggered flares when using the supplement, and there seems to be little downside to it, so it is definitely worth trying. Taking the supplement before eating a rich meal or a high-risk food may reduce the consequences. Don't use this as an excuse for lazy eating, though! Your diet still needs to eliminate the foods and drinks that exacerbate symptoms.

L-Arginine

One of the most common amino acids in the body, L-arginine is not typically taken as a supplement because our bodies produce enough of it, and it's common in many foods. L-arginine may be important for IC patients, however, because it leads to the creation of nitric oxide within the body, a molecule that opens blood vessels and increases circulation.

Researchers have noted that some patients with IC have lowered amounts of nitric oxide in their urine. In a double-blinded controlled trial, about fifty IC patients received either L-arginine or a placebo. Researchers found that overall improvement with L-arginine was 48 percent—almost double the 24 percent shown in the control group. The subjects took 1,500 mg daily over the course of three months, and improvements were noted in both pain and urgency. While exactly how it works is unknown, the study showed that L-arginine may have a modest benefit for some patients, with a low risk of side effects.

Aloe Vera

Aloe vera comes from the leaves of a cactus, and is one of the oldest known herbal remedies—it's been used for at least three millennia. Scientific evidence is mixed with respect to the benefits of aloe vera in a wide variety of conditions, but it is commonly found in cosmetics, lotions, and as an alternative medicine. It's traditionally been used to soothe burns, and research has shown there are benefits to the topical use of aloe vera on wounds.

In interstitial cystitis, it may have a different effect. Preliminary research in animal models has actually found that, when taken orally, aloe vera actually increased the production of glycosaminoglycans (GAGs) in healing wounds. Because the bladder is protected by a layer of the same substance, aloe vera may help reinforce the GAG layer in the bladder. While this theory remains unproven, it's intriguing that aloe vera might address one potential cause of IC directly at the source.

One large survey conducted by a manufacturer of concentrated aloe pills, Desert Harvest, found that 92 percent of the 600 survey respondents experienced "significant relief" with aloe vera. Although the results are not from a controlled study and should be interpreted with caution, the responses indicated that aloe vera may be able to help with urinary urgency/frequency, pelvic pain, and urethral burning. Generally, patients reported an easing of their symptoms within three months of starting treatment, so it may be worth a try for patients with IC.

Vitamin D

Vitamin D is produced naturally by the body when it's exposed to sunlight, but isn't found in many foods. It has been shown to influence bone health, but links to other health benefits have yet to be proven. A 2010 study by New York researchers found women with chronic pelvic pain, such as interstitial cystitis, were significantly more likely to have a vitamin D deficiency than the control population. Lower vitamin D levels were also correlated with an increased risk of incontinence. While it's not clear that this is a causal relationship—after all, chronic pain patients are probably less likely to be active outdoors, and are therefore more likely to be vitamin D deficient—these results, combined with the lack of vitamin D in food sources, may make the supplement an option for patients with interstitial cystitis and chronic pelvic pain. You can have your levels checked by your doctor, and can use a supplement if your levels are low.

Omega-3 Fish Oil

Two important types of omega acids have opposing effects in the body. Omega-6 fatty acids are concentrated in vegetable oils and processed foods and increase inflammation in the body. Omega-3, most commonly found in fish, reduces that inflammation. Because most Americans eat too much processed food, it's not surprising that we consume twenty times more of the former than the latter. Most experts believe that the lower the ratio of omega-6 to omega-3 fatty acids, the better.

In terms of interstitial cystitis, remember that inflammation is part of the DIP cycle (dysfunction, inflammation, pain), and you should take any opportunity to break the feedback loop. Omega-3 fish oil supplements may limit the inflammatory response from IC. And, conversely, avoiding oily or processed foods can prevent inflammation from building up. In the large ICA survey, nearly 60 percent of patients self-reported benefits from taking omega-3 supplements.

CystoProtek

One of the more popular alternative therapies for IC is a supplement combination sold under the name CystoProtek. These pills include three compounds that are building blocks of the GAG layer in the bladder, as well as two anti-inflammatory flavonoids. These supplements purport to provide the body with an additional supply of the main components of the GAG layer in the bladder, and to reduce inflammation.

CystoProtek Breakdown

CystoProtek contains the following supplements:

- Chondroitin sulfate (150 mg): An important component of cartilage and other connective tissue, chondroitin is best known as a supplement for arthritis patients. It can be absorbed into the bloodstream and distributed throughout the body, and is a primary component of the bladder GAG layer.

- Sodium hyaluronate (10 mg): This compound acts as a lubricant in joints and ligaments, and is occasionally injected into the joints of arthritis patients. It is also a component of the GAG layer in the bladder.

- Glucosamine sulfate (120 mg): Another supplement often used for arthritis, glucosamine may help the body manufacture the components of the GAG layer in the bladder.

- Quercetin (150 mg): A flavonoid found in many common foods, such as red onions, cranberries, and red apples, quercetin is thought to have anti-inflammatory properties. Quercetin has been associated with increased oxygenation of the blood and improved endurance performance in athletes.

- Rutin (20 mg): Closely related in structure and activity to quercetin, rutin is another flavonoid with demonstrated anti-inflammatory properties in animal studies.

Two surveys have been conducted with CystoProtek, but they may not be very reliable. No control group was used and the studies took place over the course of an unmonitored year, so patients taking the supplements also had various other treatments that could have had a wide range of effects on the outcome. These kinds of surveys also self-select for patients that respond well, because those seeing no benefits will often stop the treatment or not return the final survey. However, the results—whether caused by CystoProtek, the placebo effect, other treatments, or a combination—were promising. The studies reported approximately a 50 percent improvement in pain over a year of treatment with either four or six tablets of CystoProtek daily. The respondents also showed improvement in urinary symptoms.

While there is no concrete evidence that the chondroitin or sodium hyaluronate in CystoProtek reaches the bladder—or are added to the GAG layer if they do arrive—there have been documented reductions in inflammatory markers with some ingredients in CystoProtek. So, although the studies aren't conclusive, the overall results and anecdotal reports from patients indicate this combination supplement may be helpful for some people with IC. Most of its ingredients are common in other supplements and appear to be safe and tolerated well in the general population—although it does contain shellfish, to which some people are allergic. Alternatively, you can make your own regimen by purchasing the ingredients in CystoProtek individually.

Takeaways

- **Follow a healthy diet and eliminate your trigger foods.** It doesn't have to be any more complicated than that. Using a symptom log and the elimination diet, you should be able to identify personal triggers in about three months.

- **The importance of diet varies among patients.** For some patients, trigger foods are among the defining characteristics of the condition, while others find that diet has no effect on their symptoms. Most patients will be somewhere in between. Find out what effect diet has on your condition and work to make sure it's not a limiting factor for you.

- **Fuel your body for the journey.** Diet isn't just important for eliminating trigger foods: It's important to maximize your overall health on your IC journey. If you have to eliminate something from your diet, find a safe alternative to add back in. If your condition is highly food sensitive, consider consulting a nutritionist who specializes in pain conditions to find a balanced diet. Turning healthy eating into a habit should be a priority.

12

THINKING OUTSIDE THE BOX:

Nontraditional Therapies

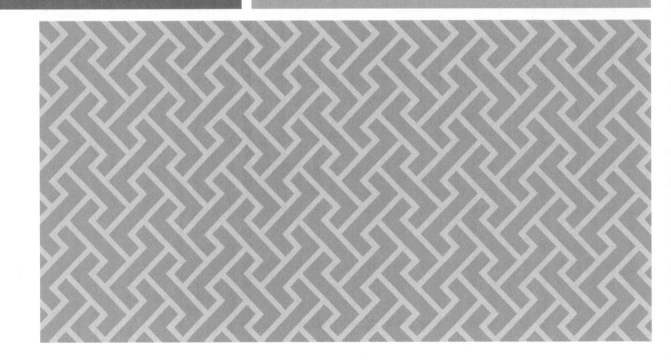

Without a clear pharmaceutical solution to interstitial cystitis, many patients look to nontraditional treatments for relief. Most alternative therapies have not been evaluated in well-conducted clinical studies, but have shown benefit for some patients in uncontrolled trials or anecdotal reports. Complementary therapies can benefit a subset of patients, and can be an important aspect of your holistic treatment plan. As with prescription medications, be wary of claims that a certain alternative therapy will completely eliminate your symptoms. This chapter guides you through some of the most popular complementary treatments for IC.

There have always been blurred lines between traditional treatments, which are widely accepted by the medical community (and now the insurance companies), and alternative therapies. Many drugs and procedures which once were solidly in the "alternative" camp have evolved into the standard of care as evidence of their benefit mounts.

Pelvic floor physical therapy was once considered an alternative treatment for pelvic floor conditions. But over the course of twenty years, rigorous studies and patient success stories have taken pelvic floor physical therapy from its status as a fringe treatment to the standard of care in IC: It is now in the first line of interventions recommended by the American Urological Association. The border between traditional and alternative treatments is fluid, constantly shifting as new evidence is brought to light; it is entirely possible that some of today's alternative treatments will be tomorrow's standard of care.

Broadly, this category is known as Complementary and Alternative Medicine (CAM). Surveys show that almost 40 percent of Americans try a nontraditional remedy each year, and these alternative treatments continue to gain popularity. Many people who explore these therapies do so for pain relief—specifically, the relief of chronic pain.

"Complementary" is the right word to describe these therapies, since they can add to—not replace—traditional treatments for interstitial cystitis. Most have not yet been evaluated in rigorous clinical trials or specifically studied for IC treatment—but we've already seen that everyone responds differently to oral medication, bladder procedures, and other traditional treatments for IC. Some patients see a lot of success with alternative treatments: So, as with any treatment, let your body be your guide. As we've discussed, there is no "right" or "wrong" way to get better. If it works for you, keep doing it.

Acupuncture

Acupuncture is among the best examples of the thin line between traditional and alternative therapy. It's been around for at least 2,000 years, spreading throughout Asia before making its way to Europe in the late 1600s. The process involves placing thin needles at very specific points over the body, typically along lines known as meridians: According to traditional Chinese medicine, energy is transferred along these lines. There are more than 400 acupuncture points. While several different theories have been proposed as to how acupuncture might work, there is no conclusive intersection between Eastern and Western medicine on the mechanism of action.

The National Institutes of Health in the United States first recommended acupuncture for some conditions in the late 1990s. Now, nearly 10 percent of Americans—twenty million in all—have tried acupuncture for various ailments and pain. About half, according to a recent government survey, reported being either "extremely" or "very" satisfied with their results, while only 18 percent were not satisfied with their treatment at all. Well more than half of Americans were willing to consider acupuncture as a treatment option.

This openness to acupuncture is based on quality science. Though we still don't understand how acupuncture works (like many of our other drugs and treatments), dozens of studies have compared acupuncture to sham procedures and found that acupuncture has significant benefits in reducing pain in a variety of conditions.

The National Institutes of Health examined twenty-nine different controlled trials that evaluated nearly 18,000 people, and determined there are concrete benefits to acupuncture. And this reduction in pain isn't related solely to the placebo effect: Fake procedures, in which needles were inserted at non-acupuncture points, didn't show the same benefits.

The benefits of acupuncture have also been tested in chronic pelvic pain patients. A 2008 study in men with chronic prostatitis (either identical or closely related to interstitial cystitis) demonstrated that 73 percent responded favorably to acupuncture. This was significantly more than the 47 percent that responded to the placebo procedure. The treatments lasted thirty minutes and were administered twice a week for a total of six weeks. Six acupuncture points were addressed around the sacral nerves that are vital to pelvic floor function. The patients maintained the improvements for the entire six months during which they were followed post-treatment.

In a follow-up study the next year, the authors found that, when combined with exercise and education about the condition, acupuncture showed a clinically significant effect in all chronic prostatitis patients.

This effect has been tested in women, as well. In an uncontrolled trial of thirty-three women with chronic pelvic pain, six weeks of acupuncture twice a week reduced or eliminated pain in twenty-nine of them. Although this study didn't have a control group that would weed out the placebo effect, the fact that so many women saw clinical benefit with acupuncture is extremely promising.

The use of acupuncture need not be limited to symptoms exclusively associated with interstitial cystitis, either. Many patients with IC also have irritable bowel syndrome or chronic constipation, and some studies have examined acupuncture's ability to treat these symptoms. Though the evidence has not concluded that acupuncture is significantly more beneficial than the sham procedure, both resulted in improvements for patients and were at least as effective as medication in one trial. Acupuncture was also shown to be effective in reducing pain and symptoms associated with menstruation.

If you decide to try acupuncture, find a licensed acupuncturist who specializes in the pelvic area. Just like doctors and physical therapists, there are specializations within acupuncture. Treatment sessions typically take about half an hour and involve the insertion of five to fifteen needles that are left in place for about twenty minutes. Don't worry, though, this procedure shouldn't be very painful. In fact, some patients report no pain at all as the very thin needles are inserted, while others feel a dull ache at the site during treatment. Also, don't expect instantaneous results. Most of the medical literature on the subject recommends a minimum of ten sessions before evaluating whether or not it helps your symptoms. If you try it, stick with it long enough to determine whether it works for you.

Meditation for IC

What if there were an IC treatment that could reduce your pain, inflammation, and anxiety while improving your overall quality of life? And what if you could reap its benefits for years to come, even after only a few weeks of treatment? It's so powerful it actually alters your mind, adding neurons to the parts of the brain that govern your emotions, happiness, and self-control. What's more, there are no side effects—and it's completely free.

If we were talking about a drug, people would line up outside pharmacies around the country to get it, but meditation has been shown to do all those things. In one study, researchers from Wake Forest University found that after just four days of meditating for twenty minutes daily, volunteers reported 40 percent less pain than those who had simply rested during the same time. Just as importantly, their perception of the unpleasantness of the pain decreased by even more—almost 60 percent. Not only did meditation reduce the pain, it also helped them cope better with the pain they *did* experience! In chronic pain patients, 65 percent had a significant reduction in pain with ten weeks of beginning meditation. Other researchers proved that meditating actually decreased the amount of inflammation at the cellular level and increased the immune system's response.

In addition to proven physical benefits, meditation can also improve mental health. Researchers from Johns Hopkins University analyzed nearly fifty studies and found that meditating reduced pain, anxiety, and depression. In fact, they concluded meditation was just as effective against depression as antidepressant medication—but without the side effects and cost. After only two months of meditation, depressed volunteers reported significant improvements in their anxiety and depressive symptoms, and these improvements continued for three years beyond the initial study

So why aren't more of us meditating? We know it has positive effects, but we don't make it part of our daily lives. This may be due, in part, to misconceptions about meditation. You don't need to sit cross-legged in an incense-filled room or be cloistered in a Tibetan monastery to get its benefits. In fact, after finding it improved emotional, mental, and physical performance, the United States military is training soldiers in meditation techniques. Professional athletes meditate to calm their minds and sharpen their abilities. There are dozens of different types of meditation; there is certainly one for you.

Guided Imagery

Guided imagery is a meditation technique that has shown a moderate effect on the pain and symptoms of IC patients. Primarily a relaxation technique that prompts patients to imagine various soothing sensations, guided imagery takes the focus off pain and symptoms with these images. In a controlled clinical trial with thirty IC patients, a 15 percent improvement was noted in both pain and general symptoms—almost identical to the control group results. The patients had to commit significant amounts of time to the intervention, since they were asked to listen to a thirty-minute CD twice daily for a total of eight weeks. The greatest benefit was seen in the frequency of urination, which decreased from sixteen to twelve times daily in the guided imagery group. While some patients did respond favorably to the treatment, other techniques may offer better results in exchange for the time investment. However, many people find guided imagery soothing and comforting; if you've tried it and it works for you, stick with it.

Cognitive-Behavioral Therapy

Cognitive-behavioral therapy (CBT) is a form of psychotherapy that focuses on restoring a sense of control to patients. Behavioral therapy attempts to change habits, encourage positive traits, and reduce negative actions, while cognitive therapy has the same goal for thought patterns. Cognitive-behavioral therapy combines these two disciplines, helping patients develop positive mental and physical habits that improve overall health. Creating healthy habits means you don't need to rely exclusively on your willpower; they become as routine as brushing your teeth or tying your shoes.

This therapy can be a powerful tool. CBT was shown to be superior to antidepressants in fighting depressive symptoms. It's highly effective in managing the anxiety and catastrophizing that can be associated with chronic pain conditions, such as interstitial cystitis.

But CBT isn't just meant to make you feel better or give you a more positive outlook on life. Clinical trials have proven it significantly reduces pain and symptoms in a number of chronic conditions, including cancer, chronic lower back pain, and pelvic pain. Interestingly, cognitive-behavioral therapy was shown to reduce both the actual amount of pain experienced and how well patients dealt with the pain they did feel.

Chronic pain patients who tried even a few sessions of CBT reported less disability and were able to increase their daily activities. Their visits to doctors and other healthcare providers became less frequent, since they became able to handle more of their medical concerns with self-care.

One very important study illustrates how effective cognitive-behavioral therapy can be for chronic pelvic pain. In research from Yale University published in 2009, pelvic pain patients were given ten one-hour training sessions with CBT. The training focused on two specific areas: self-management, in which patients were given specific techniques to help take care of their physical condition, and cognitive skills, helping identify and self-correct catastrophizing thoughts to regain control of their mental health.

The results were striking. On average, patients given the CBT training saw more than a 50 percent reduction in pain. These were patients who had struggled for more than six months, and who weren't helped by multiple treatments and medications. But just a few hours of learning to take control of their own health cut their pain in half within three months.

Plus, the benefits went beyond pain reduction. The women who received cognitive-behavioral therapy saw a 38 percent improvement in sexual function, another primary complaint of pelvic pain patients. Depressive symptoms and anxiety were also reduced. Even a year after the training, the patients maintained their gains—or even continued to improve. In just a few sessions of CBT training, it appears that these patients experienced lasting, significant improvements.

With CBT, patients learn about appropriate goal setting for their personal situations. The goals need to be concrete, so it's clear when they have been met. They should also be realistic and build upon each other until they accomplish the ultimate objective. By setting and meeting observable, achievable goals, you take responsibility for your recovery and focus on the aspects of healing within your control.

Cognitive-behavioral therapy works to give patients tools for their own care and a feeling of control over their medical situation; doctors, researchers, and patients are all realizing self-care can be one of the most important factors in healing from chronic conditions, such as interstitial cystitis.

Supportive Psychotherapy

In the same study that evaluated CBT in chronic pelvic pain, the authors evaluated the benefits of supportive psychotherapy. They separated it from the specific advice and training of CBT. The therapist who ran the session would simply ask the patient about how their week had gone and about their chronic pain. Therapists were specifically forbidden from providing any suggestions, interventions, or thoughts about changing patients' habits. Instead, they were trained to be accepting, nonjudgmental, and empathetic—essentially, good listeners. The therapy visits reduced pain by nearly one-third and depressive symptoms by 20 percent.

Seeing a professional therapist can be an important step. You can improve your coping mechanisms and actually reduce your pain by working with a mental health professional. There are experts within the field who specialize in challenging pain conditions. Some patients see a psychologist for just a few visits after their diagnosis to set them on the right track; others make visits to a counselor a regular part of their IC journey.

Takeaways

- **Alternative treatments should be complementary.** The treatments in this chapter may be of benefit, but have not been as rigorously evaluated as most traditional therapies. They shouldn't replace more traditional treatments. Use your symptom log to see whether one or more is effective for you.

- **Don't discount the idea that a complementary treatment can work for you.** While the research is limited for many alternative treatments for IC, pilot studies and patient reports indicate these treatments may offer benefits. In general, there's little downside to trying some, and there may be substantial upside. Again, they shouldn't replace traditional treatments, but they can be part of a holistic treatment approach on your IC journey.

- **Mental and emotional health is just as important as physical health.** It can reduce IC symptoms, increase your energy, and improve your quality of life by changing how you think about your condition. Investing in your mental health via meditation or traditional therapy can reap huge dividends, and should be thought of as an essential part of a holistic treatment routine.

SECTION III

The Three Stages of
Recovery: Your Action Plan

13

STAGE I:
Manage the Symptoms

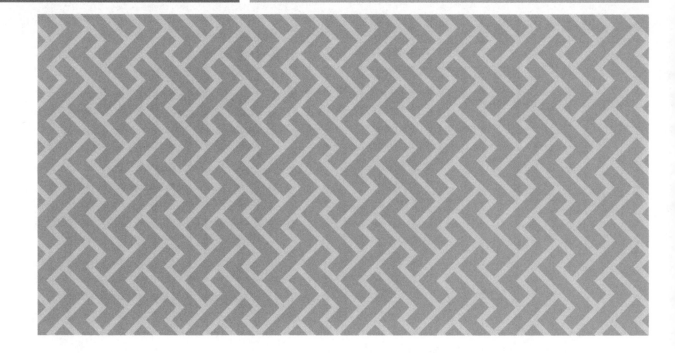

Now that you have the information about interstitial cystitis and your treatment options, the challenge is to integrate it into your daily life to see real, sustained improvement. To do that, it's helpful to think of your recovery in three discrete stages. The time you spend in each stage can vary, but you'll need to graduate from all of them to reach your destination. Have faith in yourself: You can and, with perseverance, you will, reach these milestones.

At each stage, you'll have a goal for each category of treatment. It's natural to be more comfortable with some treatments than with others, but all play an important role. Don't neglect a certain type of treatment just because you aren't as familiar with it.

Remember: These are general guidelines and recommendations. Everyone with interstitial cystitis is different, and you need to tailor your program to fit your own condition, ability level, and the amount of time you are able to invest in your recovery. Listen to your doctors, your physical therapist, and—above all—your own body.

The most important thing, whether you have just been diagnosed with IC or have battled the condition for years, is to act. There are many ways to recover—as many ways as there are patients with IC—but all require an investment of time and energy in your health. Take the first step toward healing.

Take First Steps

During Stage I, you'll begin to understand interstitial cystitis, both the general condition and your individual case. You'll realize you have the power to effect change. And you'll work to seize control of your health and to discover (or rediscover) a hope of recovery.

You'll also be challenged to keep an open mind. If you've struggled with IC for years, you'll need to let go of some of your preconceptions: If you're just starting your IC journey, there's a lot to learn. You may be uncomfortable with some treatments outlined in this book. Perhaps you've been taught that IC is exclusively a bladder condition and have based your treatment decisions on that assumption for years. In that case, it may be hard to accept that physical therapy, stretching, or stress management can be among your most powerful tools. By keeping an open mind, you'll maximize your ability to find the best treatments for you.

As you discover which treatments are most beneficial, you'll begin to see change. It may be small at first, but you'll be able to continue building on those gains. Keeping your symptom log to track your progress should be a habit. Gradual change and improvement can be hard to see when you're in the trenches. The symptom log (chapter 2) lets you stand back and view the bigger picture. Having an objective history is a map of your journey, allowing you to see how far you've come and what's propelling your recovery.

Oral Medications: Observe the Benefits and Side Effects

Whether just diagnosed or working to control your interstitial cystitis for a long time, oral medications can be very important. They can help reduce pain, calm your nervous system, prevent inflammation, and relax tight muscles. As discussed in chapter 7, there are many options.

When it comes to which oral medications to try first, let your symptoms be your guide. If pain is your primary complaint—and especially if you've been in pain for a long time—focus on relieving your discomfort. An antidepressant, which can calm your nervous system, is a logical option, particularly if you have exhibited any signs of depression. An antihistamine can help with the inflammation associated with IC, and also has benefits in treating allergies or heartburn. Many patients find success trying oral medications in several categories to get the maximum benefit, especially early on in treatment. Plus, many of these can be over-the-counter medications instead of prescriptions, especially antihistamines. For those in such pain that daily activities are impossible, opioid painkillers, medical marijuana, or other pain management medication may be necessary until you can reduce your symptoms. Tell your doctor about all medications you're taking, even nonprescription drugs.

ORAL MEDICATION CHART

Oral medication	Date started	Length of time to effect*	Observed benefits	Observed side effects

Use this chart to keep track of your medications. A summary can be helpful for you as well as your medical team. Note when you start a new treatment, and how long it's supposed to take for the medication to work. For example, antidepressants often take at least three weeks to begin to show an effect, while PPS can take six months. See chapter 7, and ask your doctor how long the medication should take to show a benefit.

Use your medication chart in conjunction with your symptom log to evaluate how well you respond to these medications. Part of your interstitial cystitis journey is learning which treatments deliver the most benefit while minimizing unpleasant side effects.

Bladder Treatments: Decide Whether Bladder Instillations Help

When you try bladder instillations, it will quickly become apparent whether they will be successful reducing your symptoms. If they do, each treatment will provide between three and ten days of pain relief, and may help with urgency and frequency of urination. Continue these treatments throughout this first stage: They will reduce the dysfunction–inflammation–pain (DIP) cycle and give your body a respite from the constant symptoms of interstitial cystitis.

If bladder instillations do not provide symptom relief, or if the catheterization procedure causes too much irritation to continue, consider neuromodulation. Percutaneous tibial nerve stimulation (PTNS) is a non-invasive procedure shown to be effective in relieving pain and bladder symptoms. A trial of neuromodulation involves one treatment weekly for three months, so you should learn relatively quickly whether it will be of benefit.

Pelvic Floor Physical Therapy: Schedule an Evaluation

As we've seen, pelvic floor physical therapy is the only treatment shown to sustainably help the majority of IC patients. The first step is to find a qualified, experienced pelvic floor PT. A few therapy sessions should let you know whether there's a strong pelvic floor component to your pain and symptoms: If the PT is able to reproduce your IC symptoms with internal or external trigger points, then the pelvic floor is a factor. As discussed in chapter 9, you should see a change in symptoms in the first four to six visits. If your current pelvic floor PT isn't able to reproduce your symptoms, or you don't see a change in your first six visits, consider getting a second opinion.

Self-Care: Start a Daily Routine

One unique aspect of IC treatment is that you can achieve significant improvement in symptoms with self-care. In this first stage of treatment, begin with the complete stretching program in chapter 10. This should take less than thirty minutes daily. If finding the time is challenging, you can multitask and do stretching while you watch TV, talk on the phone, or before bed.

Work on deep breathing as you stretch, which helps relax the pelvic floor and calms the entire body. Many patients make this a time of quiet meditation, incorporating breathing techniques from mindfulness meditation or yoga. Get into the habit of taking a daily walk, too. When you first start, you might walk for just five minutes along a flat path—that's fine. Exercise, sunshine, and fresh air have major benefits.

This is also a good time to do gentle self-massage, working on fascial and trigger point release. Begin with your abdomen, and notice how much better the area feels after you spend a few minutes doing fascial release. You can then move down to your inner and upper thighs, feeling the tension leave the muscles as you clear them of dysfunction. These areas may be tender and painful when you start, so give yourself permission to go slowly. If you're going to pelvic floor physical therapy, let your therapist observe your self-care techniques to make sure you are doing them properly.

Diet: Eliminate Common Culprits

As you've read, diet is a major component of successfully managing interstitial cystitis. Nearly 90 percent of patients with IC report changes in their symptoms with what they eat and drink. You don't need major changes in your diet to start; begin by eliminating some of the most common triggers. As you do, note how your body responds in your symptom log: It's important to determine early on in your IC journey whether or not you're highly food sensitive. Start with eliminating these items:

- Alcoholic and carbonated beverages
- Artificial sweeteners
- Caffeine
- Citrus fruits and juices
- Spicy and exotic foods
- Tomatoes and tomato-based foods

To sustainably remove these foods and drinks from your diet, it's important to find ways to replace them with similar, nontrigger foods. Switch your morning cup of coffee to herbal tea, or use a white sauce instead of marinara on pasta. Get creative—take a cooking class with your partner, or make a weekly meal plan and shopping list. If you struggle with IBS, consider cutting dairy out of your diet for several weeks to see how it affects your symptoms.

Keep a list of "safe foods"—the ones you're completely confident in—along with your list of trigger foods. When in doubt, use these safe foods to make healthy choices.

Alternative and Complementary Treatments: Try Something New

There are many alternative supplements and treatments you can try in Stage I. Again, let your symptoms and past experience guide you. For example, if you've had success with acupuncture for another type of pain, consider visiting an acupuncturist who specializes in the pelvis.

Some patients are already on a supplement regimen that includes omega-3 fish oil or vitamin D, both of which may be beneficial for IC patients. For those who are highly food sensitive, the antacid calcium glycerophosphate (Prelief) may be useful to take with meals. L-arginine, aloe vera, CystoProtek, and other supplements have major proponents in the IC community. In this first stage, try something new, and use your symptom log to track whether it has benefit for you.

Mental Health: Relieve Stress and Relax the Nervous System

Concentrating on your mental health can be a vital part of your recovery. Emotional health is important for everyone, and working to develop it will be a major part of your journey.

In this first stage, focus on relieving stress and relaxing the nervous system. Practice deep breathing, focusing on the rise and fall of your breath. Let your anxiety fade away with each exhale. If you have experience with meditation or yoga, this may be the time to revisit those exercises. Identify any underlying sources of emotional distress and work to address them. Start with these home exercises, but if you need more support, consider an appointment with a psychologist or other specialist.

Solving the Puzzle versus Regaining Your Life—Which Is More Important?

This book suggests you try many things at once to address your IC symptoms, and then observe which ones result in improvement. This contrasts with the way many doctors prefer to work. Doctors often view interstitial cystitis as a puzzle: The best way to solve it is to introduce one treatment at a time and evaluate how your symptoms respond. If you try two or more things at the same time, the reasoning goes, you won't know which one is really responsible for your improvement.

Unfortunately, this step-by-step approach can take a long time to result in meaningful improvements. For instance, it may take six months before the doctor is convinced that the first oral medication she prescribed isn't effective or not effective enough. She'll then take you off the medication and switch you to a new one. If that doesn't give the hoped-for improvement, maybe you'll be referred to physical therapy or given still another drug. All the while the condition is worsening and the DIP cycle is active, making it more difficult to calm your nervous system when you do find effective treatment.

Often, the answer is a combination of therapies anyway, so taking extra time to try them one at a time is difficult to justify, and leads to additional physical and mental consequences from dealing with the pain and symptoms while you gather clues.

Even if you do try each medication or treatment one at a time, you still can't be positive that it's responsible for the difference you notice. Dozens of factors influence IC symptoms: diet, exercise, posture, the pelvic floor, constipation, sex, depression, physical activities, stress, anxiety, catastrophizing, associated conditions, and other processes happening within the body on a microscopic level, such as inflammation and neural regulation. With all those elements, it's nearly impossible to identify one medication or treatment conclusively as being responsible for improvement.

If you don't get better on a medication, the doctor will assume it's because the medication isn't working. But what if the medication *is* working? What if you'd be much worse without it? Maybe you have a lot of stress in your life; your irritable bowel syndrome has acted up, your diet is out of control, and you aren't exercising. In this case, perhaps the medication is the only thing keeping your symptoms from being far worse than they could be! On the other hand, if you show improvement on a certain drug, is the improvement due to the drug itself? Or, are you just taking better care of yourself, too? Do everything in your power to see improvement immediately; don't suffer while trying to solve an impossible puzzle.

Before graduating from Stage I, you need a check mark by all the items in the chart on the next page.

CHARTING YOUR RECOVERY

	Stage I: Manage Your Symptoms	✓	Stage II: Address Underlying Issues	Stage III: Living Successfully with IC
Oral medication	Start medication, observe benefits and side effects			
Bladder treatments	Try bladder instillations			
Pelvic floor PT	Try pelvic floor PT and determine how much your pelvic floor contributes to your pain			
Self-care	Begin daily stretching regimen; work on fascial and trigger point release			
Diet	Eliminate the most common problem foods with interstitial cystitis; determine level of food sensitivity			
Complementary treatments	Try something new			
Mental health	Work to relieve stress and relax the nervous system; practice deep breathing; identify underlying sources of emotional distress			
Goals	Take action; see a change in your condition, and learn what your IC responds best to			

Takeaways

- **Take first steps.** When recovering from IC, knowledge really is power. Understanding the condition gives you control over your health and the power to make lasting changes. Use your symptom log and the information in this book to demystify your condition. You have all the information, now it's time to act.

- **Assemble your tools for the journey.** Successfully treating IC requires a holistic approach. There are complex interactions with the condition, and no single treatment or technique will carry you to your destination. In Stage I, identify the most important tools for your unique IC journey.

- **See a change.** This is the stage at which you'll first see a change in your symptoms. This change may be slight or substantial, but it should be there if you follow the plan. Note the differences you see as you begin treatments, and learn what will be important in your continued recovery. The time you take in this stage can vary, but it is typically around three to six months for most patients. Remember to try different treatments at the same time; a holistic treatment regimen will be necessary, and the sooner you can see a change, the better.

For New and Veteran Patients

If you are new to IC, this can be an overwhelming time. It may seem as if there are too many pieces of the puzzle, and you're having trouble seeing what the finished picture will look like. You may be working to find a quality medical team (see page 189) and trying to find doctors and other medical practitioners who are the right fit for you.

For you, it's important to just get on the path and start walking. Take first steps. You'll start to find treatments that work best for you, and the pieces will start to fall into place.

If you're an IC veteran, this is your opportunity to look at your condition with fresh eyes. The challenge is to make use of your experience, but still be open to new ideas. There will be first steps for you as well in this stage. You may be pushed to find a new path, or you may need to reevaluate treatments that you tried before with the new knowledge that you've gained. Listen to your body, and trust that there are treatments out there that will benefit your unique condition.

14

STAGE II:
Address Underlying Issues

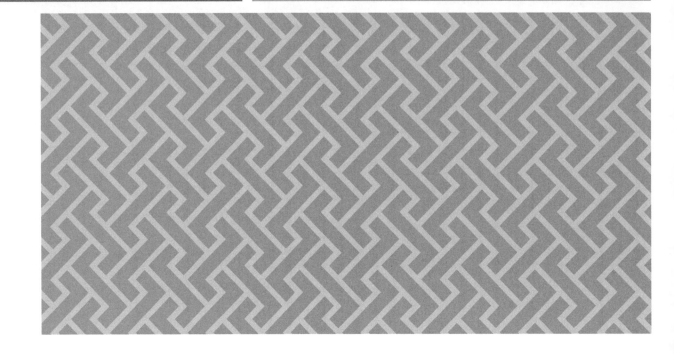

Congratulations on graduating from Stage I. In Stage II, you'll fine-tune your treatments and healing regimen. You'll develop concrete goals about family, work, exercise, and other activities. You've already learned how your body responds to different treatments, so now you can focus on the most beneficial ones.

This is also the part of the path that can be the most difficult to follow. In the early days of your treatment, you often see a relatively rapid improvement in some of your symptoms. In this stage, you'll realize your recovery is really a journey. Your improvement will continue, but it won't always take a straight path—and, sometimes, even feel like you're going in the wrong direction. But it's essential, more now than ever, that you lace up your boots each morning and stay the course.

During this stage of your recovery you'll be challenged to dig deep and to address any underlying issues holding you back. For some patients, this is the bladder itself, which can seem like an intractable enemy. For others, pelvic floor dysfunction is the major barrier to healing. Maintaining a healthy diet may not yet be a habit, and can be a struggle. Some patients discover buried emotional barriers that prevent progress. Whatever your personal roadblock is, you'll be challenged to press ahead with treatment and remove it from your path.

This time can also be exciting—you're beginning to regain your life. As your physical condition improves, you'll have to make some smart decisions about your daily activities. Often, activity level and symptoms rise or fall together. Treatment can keep symptoms at a manageable level as you increase your activity, but there can be a trade-off if you overdo it. Be gentle with yourself, and make sure your body responds well as you return to regular activities.

A Word on Willpower

We've all had the experience. December 31, motivated and ready to change, we pledge to lose those extra pounds, call our mothers more often, and finally learn to play that dusty guitar in the closet. And we really mean it! Yet, most of us will make the very same resolutions next year. Why?

Here's the answer. Scientists have discovered that willpower is a finite resource. We have this mistaken belief that if we just put our minds to something, we can do it. But instead, we're learning that willpower is limited, and can be used up if we try to do too much.

In one of the best experiments proving this theory, researchers brought in volunteers to take a series of tests. They put a plate of delicious cookies and a bowl of unappetizing radishes on the table. Some people were asked to resist temptation and eat only the radishes, while others were allowed to eat as many cookies as they wanted. Then each volunteer was asked to attempt a mental exercise that was impossible: Researchers wanted to see how long volunteers would use their willpower to continue to work on the puzzle.

What happened? Those who had used willpower to avoid the cookies quit twice as early as those who allowed themselves to indulge! This result redefined the way in which we think about willpower. After all, if some people "just have a lot of willpower," why would having to choose between radishes and cookies affect their perseverance in a totally unrelated activity? Because they had dipped into their willpower reserve to resist the cookies, they had less left to fight to complete the exercise.

"If you create one healthy habit each month, at the end of the year, you'd have twelve new tools for your IC journey!"

So, how do you use this information in your IC journey?

1. Stop wasting willpower on things that don't matter. Your IC journey is going to require a lot of your energy, so focus on what is most important. Prioritize your health; don't spend your valuable willpower elsewhere.

2. Turn chores into habits. How much willpower do you spend each morning deciding to brush your teeth? None. It's part of your routine. As activities become habits, they no longer require decisions and willpower. And research has shown that developing a habit only takes about twenty-one days. Once you transform an activity into a habit, you no longer expend energy to make it happen.

One great example with my patients is stretching. At first, it's a challenge and requires active willpower—but after about a month, it's a natural part of their day. Maybe it's the first thing they do when they roll out of bed. Or, instead of sitting on the couch to watch TV at the end of the day, they sit on the floor and stretch. And it all adds up: If you create one healthy habit each month, at the end of the year, you'd have twelve new tools for your IC journey!

Oral Medication:
Optimize Your Medications

As you learn which oral medications are effective in reducing pain and urinary symptoms, you'll be able to fine-tune your medications. This often involves finding the correct dosage, which provides clinical benefit but reduces adverse effects of the drugs. Sometimes this will mean switching to a new version of a drug, or finding a generic that fits within your budget.

You may also add new medications during this part of your journey. Perhaps your nervous system has been calmed by an antidepressant medication, but you also want to see if an antihistamine can provide further benefits.

This is not the time to eliminate medications. You should focus on regaining your life and functional activities with your medications intact. Once you reach your goals, you can taper off or eliminate certain drugs, while making sure your condition remains the same. Many patients are uncomfortable taking long-term medication, but this is not the time to upset the delicate balance you worked hard to create.

Bladder Treatments: Bladder Instillations and Other Options

As with oral medications, this stage is an opportunity for you to perfect your bladder treatments. Find a bladder treatment that provides symptom relief during this stage, even if you decide only to use it during flares. If bladder instillations work for you, continue to use them to decrease pain and frequency. This will give you an advantage in every other aspect as you continue your recovery.

If you haven't done so already, this is definitely the time to try percutaneous tibial nerve stimulation (PTNS). Treatments stretch over a twelve-week span, and you should be able to find a local doctor to administer them. If the less-invasive PTNS neuromodulation isn't working, you may want to explore the surgical alternative with the sacral nerve.

If you are in the minority of IC patients with Hunner's lesions, they can be removed from the bladder to relieve pain. If these treatments haven't provided the desired improvement, it may now be appropriate to consider intradetrusor BOTOX for the first time and to determine whether it is beneficial for you.

Pelvic Floor Physical Therapy: Work on the "Why"

Assuming you're among the 90 percent of patients aided by pelvic floor physical therapy, this part of your journey will involve determining and addressing the specific underlying causes of your dysfunction. Your urethral muscles might be constantly strained and tight. The pelvis can be out of alignment, or there may be a nagging tailbone injury or low back pain holding back your recovery.

Your pelvic floor PT should be able to identify your primary issues and why they exist. Once you know the causes, you can focus on eliminating these limiting factors.

As you figure out the "why" of your condition, your treatment sessions and home program can alleviate the underlying problems. When these major trigger points or stresses are released, your entire pelvic floor will begin to function properly again. You'll feel the pelvic floor component of your interstitial cystitis ease, and you'll note a reduction in symptoms. Breaking the cycle of bladder problems and pelvic floor dysfunction allows true healing to take place.

"A nutritionist can help you develop a healthy eating plan that's free from your personal triggers."

Self-Care: Tailor Your Pelvic Floor Regimen

Now that you are comfortable with your stretching routine, you should notice your muscles releasing the tension they carry, relaxing more easily. The fascial release you began in Stage I should begin to clear up some inflammation trapped underneath the skin, and you should be more confident in your fascial release techniques.

You may have started trigger point release, especially externally, but, in this stage, trigger point release will become instrumental in improving your pelvic floor and surrounding muscles. A foam roller can make external trigger point release easier. Remember always to follow your trigger point release with stretching to help prevent knots from returning.

While you continue to address external trigger points, add internal trigger point release to your routine during this part of your journey. In this stage, you'll become expert at finding and releasing these trigger points, thereby eliminating the pelvic floor dysfunction contributing to your pain and urgency. Your knowledge of your pelvic floor will allow you to move directly to points that hold tension and cause symptoms, and clear them quickly to reduce symptoms.

Diet: Take the Next Step

At this stage, the path diverges for many patients. After eliminating most of the obvious culprits, some patients determine they're not highly food sensitive. If you don't notice a major benefit to your IC symptoms after removing the top five trigger foods, you can add back some of those foods—but make sure they don't flare your symptoms. Add them one at a time, over the course of a week. By following this elimination diet, you determine which specific categories cause problems and can avoid only those foods.

Some patients will find they are highly food sensitive. If eliminating the common trigger foods has a dramatic impact on your health, you may feel there might be additional foods and beverages holding you back. In that case, use your symptom log and the ICA food list to selectively eliminate other foods that may flare symptoms. Once you see improvement in your symptoms, add foods back into your diet, one at a time, to determine which ones were your individual triggers.

If you are highly food sensitive, it's important to add new foods to your diet to compensate for the ones you've eliminated. A nutritionist can help you develop a healthy eating plan that's free from your personal triggers.

Whether or not you're highly food sensitive, planning your meals for the week can make it easier to stick with your diet. Involve your family, and make this a habit during this stage.

Alternative and Complementary Treatments: Add Something to Your Treatment

You've already tried at least one alternative or complementary therapy in Stage I. If it was successful, make sure it remains a consistent part of your routine.

If the first one you tried wasn't effective, now is your chance to try something new. There are many options in this category, and it's almost certain that one can have a positive impact on your condition. Continue to explore until you find something that works for you, then make sure to incorporate it into your holistic treatment regimen.

Mental Health: Delve Deeper

This is the part of your journey where your mental health becomes even more important. When you first find an effective treatment and feel relief, you might feel an initial burst of excitement. But that energy can fade during this stage, since your results might be less dramatic: You're more likely to experience incremental improvements, and even the occasional setback. That can be frustrating, but don't give in to catastrophizing or negative thoughts. It's vital to continue your mental health exercises from Stage I, whether deep breathing, meditation, yoga, or seeing a professional. Take an objective look at the stressors in your life and how you react to them. The benefits of removing stress from your system are many and crucial to a successful recovery.

Now is the time to dig deeply into any underlying issues impeding your journey to health. Be honest about your emotional state, and decide whether professional help might be beneficial. If not, make sure you have another way—a supportive partner or friend, consistent meditation, cognitive-behavioral therapy, or other method—to develop positive mental habits.

Goal Setting: Creating Signposts

To get where you want to be on your IC journey, you need signposts and markers along the way. The destination can seem distant, but breaking the journey into small goals makes each day manageable.

Your goals are personal, and are very important to guide your healing. Be honest with yourself when you set these milestones. For example, you may have to prioritize which of your symptoms are the most problematic for you. Should your treatment focus on reducing pain, or are urinary symptoms having a larger effect on your life? Is regaining a sexual relationship with your partner high on your list of goals, or is returning to work a more immediate priority? Different goals might lead you to different treatment options.

Start by formulating your big-picture goals. Your overall goal might be to return to work or your daily activities, even with lingering symptoms. Keep that end in mind as you set smaller goals that will lead you to it.

SMART Goals

Make sure your goals are SMART—specific, measurable, achievable, relevant, and timely.

Specific goals clearly identify what you want to accomplish.

Measurable goals have an objective way to know if you achieve them.

Attainable goals push and stretch you, but can be achieved.

Relevant goals relate to your big-picture goal and build toward it.

Timely goals have a specific target date for achievement: They aren't indefinite.

Focus on the Process

Whenever possible, your goals should be process oriented rather than results oriented. To be attainable, they need to be something you can control. Obviously, your ultimate aim is to reduce your symptoms, but you can't control how quickly your body responds to treatment, especially in the beginning when you don't yet know which treatments are most effective for you. So, setting a goal to reduce pain or return to work by the end of the month can be counterproductive; meeting that goal may not be within your power. It may take your body longer to heal, even if you do everything right. However, if your goal relates to the healing process, it remains entirely in your control.

Many patients find that weekly or monthly checklists are great tools. A visual representation of your process can be a powerful motivator. Create one of your own, use the one following, or use the online template at PelvicSanity.com.

Results Oriented	Process Oriented
See a reduction in my pain symptoms	Spend 30 minutes each day doing stretches and self-care and log my activity.
Reduce my urinary frequency	Keep track of my urinary symptoms with a bladder diary, and determine which treatments are successful in reducing urgency and frequency.
Stop feeling so anxious and stressed	Meditate each day, and set a timer to remind myself to take deep breaths each hour.
Take medication to eliminate my bladder pain	Try the medication for 1 month and keep a detailed symptom log to understand whether it helps, and note any side effects I experience.

Choose process-oriented goals.

SAMPLE CHECKLIST

Goal	Mon	Tues	Wed	Thur	Fri	Sat	Sun
20 minutes of stretching							
Meditate							
Take medications							
Eat a healthy diet							
Internal trigger point release							
Other:							
Other:							

CHARTING YOUR RECOVERY

	Stage I: Manage Your Symptoms	Stage II: Address Underlying Issues	✓	Stage III: Living Successfully with IC
Oral medication	Start medication, observe benefits, and side effects	Fine-tune medications to increase benefits and reduce side effects		
Bladder treatments	Try bladder instillations	If bladder instillations are not effective, try neurostimulation or behavioral training		
Pelvic floor PT	Try pelvic floor PT and determine how much your pelvic floor contributes to your pain	Continue with pelvic floor PT; work on the "why"—figure out underlying causes and work to address them		
Self-care	Begin daily stretching regimen; work on fascial and trigger point release	Tailor stretching and strengthening to your specific problem areas; become comfortable with internal and external trigger point release at home		
Diet	Eliminate the most common problem foods with IC and determine level of food sensitivity	Take the next step with your diet: add foods back in or find additional trigger foods to remove		
Complementary treatments	Try something new	Add something to your daily regimen		
Mental health	Work to relieve stress and relax the nervous system; practice deep breathing; identify underlying sources of emotional distress	Actively work on your mental health: consider meditation, cognitive-behavioral therapy, a psychologist, or an IC support group		
Goals	Take action; see a change in your condition, and learn what your IC responds best to	Develop specific goals for your recovery; keep going, and stay positive through bumps in the road		

Takeaways

- **Stay the course.** During Stage II, you may be disappointed with the lack of immediate benefit. Don't give up hope. The time and energy you put toward your recovery are investments in your future health. You may not see dramatic, overnight improvements, but you will eventually look back on this time as essential in your road to recovery.

- **Keep the destination in mind.** The goals you set during this time should be realistic and attainable. They should recognize your current limitations, but still be filled with hope for the future. Be honest with yourself, and determine what's most important to you. Communicate these goals to your medical professionals, your friends, and your family. Knowing where you want to go will get you there more quickly.

For New and Veteran Patients

If you are a new patient with IC, don't be discouraged by your first major setback or the small, daily fluctuations in your symptoms. Though you still may have good days and bad days, you should be noticing a trend toward recovery. This is one of the reasons it is important to keep a good symptom log; even on tough days, you can look back and see exactly how far you have come. What you are now experiencing as a "bad day" might have been your best day just a few short months ago. Disappointment is the enemy; keep your eyes on your goal and stay the course through this stage.

If you are a veteran patient, you may feel like you've been at this stage before—and you probably have. Trust the process and keep putting one foot in front of the other. Don't allow frustration to lead to inaction at this critical stage when you need to push through. You may need to dig deeper, in one area or another, to break through walls that are holding you back. Some plateaus are inevitable, but keep your focus on the destination.

15

STAGE III:

Living Successfully with IC

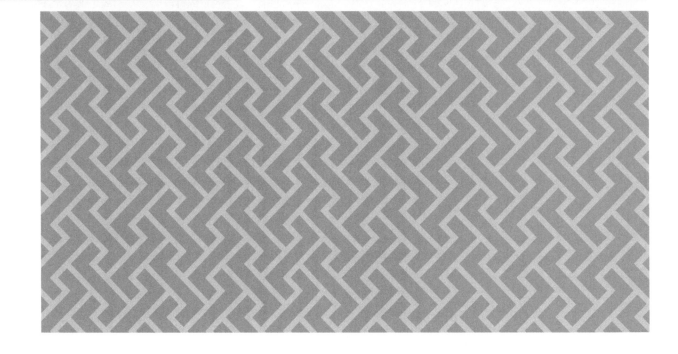

This is the final stretch of your IC journey. You've begun a variety of treatments and have identified the unique areas you need to address to heal. You have created a holistic and multi-disciplinary treatment regimen, and have seen marked improvements in your symptoms. Now you need to hold onto the progress you've made, while regaining control of your life.

In Stage 3, your approach shifts from striving for improvement to maintaining your gains. Now that your symptoms are manageable—perhaps they haven't disappeared completely, but are greatly improved—you know what your body needs to keep your IC under control. Healthy lifestyle choices, such as stretching, self-care, avoiding prolonged sitting, and following a balanced diet, should be habits. You know the pros and cons of each different treatment option, and you have created a sustainable, holistic regimen that works for you.

A major goal of this phase is to be confident in dealing with the occasional symptom flare when it happens. You'll create a detailed plan, so you'll know exactly what to do when one strikes. And you'll probably be able to recognize what led to the flare: Going off your diet, prolonged sitting, neglecting your self-care regimen, a change in medication, or an emotional stressor can all contribute to a flare. Understanding what led to the flare and having a plan to deal with it can give you the confidence to manage your health effectively when one occurs.

With your symptoms under control and a system in place for dealing with flares, this can be a time of restoration. Test your limits. See how your body responds as you experiment with new activities. Whether you call this period remission, recovery, or management, it's when you get to celebrate your journey and be proud of how far you've come.

Oral Medications: Your Maintenance Regimen

Your goal now is to return to your normal life while minimizing your use of prescription drugs. In this final stage, the challenge is to find a permanent regimen that allows you to have minimal symptoms at your desired level of activity. Some patients don't require any prescription medication once their symptoms are under control, while others benefit greatly from ongoing treatment. Your program is unique to you, and, by now, you have discovered which medications deliver the most benefit with the fewest side effects. Once you reach your desired level of activity—whether that's going back to work, returning to daily exercise, or being more involved with your family—you can establish which medications you need to maintain that lifestyle.

For many people, this means weaning themselves off drugs that were an essential part of their journey. Now that your symptoms are manageable and you've addressed some underlying issues of the condition, you may no longer need all your oral medications. Breakthrough pain or flares can be managed when they arise, either with a prescription or over-the-counter medication. Talk to your doctor about decreasing your medications gradually and safely when you're ready. Find the lowest dose that still provides benefit. If you do notice an unacceptable increase in symptoms when reducing your oral medications, don't be afraid to return to an earlier, more effective dosage, and reassess your plan.

Bladder Treatments: Decide How They Fit

By now you'll know whether bladder treatments are an integral part of your holistic treatment plan. Many patients begin with regular bladder instillations to treat the immediate pain and symptoms of the condition, but can gradually reduce the frequency as their condition improves. If they're effective for you, these treatments can be saved for times when symptoms flare and you need an additional intervention.

If bladder instillations continue to be an important part of your treatment plan, you can administer these yourself, saving both time and money. Learning to self-catheterize allows you to use the treatments on your own schedule, and opens up the possibility of travel and more freedom from doctor visits.

You may have also tried neurostimulation. Protocols for tibial nerve stimulation recommend a maintenance procedure once a month to keep the gains you have made. If you have had a sacral nerve stimulator implanted, keep in contact with the manufacturer's representative. Your program can be changed to provide more relief during a flare, and may be modified if it becomes less effective over time.

If urinary symptoms are still a concern, this is a great time to try bladder training, if you haven't already. By gradually increasing the amount of time between voids, you can retrain your bladder to reduce urinary frequency (see chapter 10 for more information). You'll also need to decide whether to continue other bladder procedures if you have found them effective. Hunner's lesions tend to reoccur; if you experienced pain relief after having yours removed, schedule a regular checkup with your doctor. If you found success with BOTOX to the bladder, the usual

course is to have the procedure repeated every six months. Once you've had success with BOTOX, you can allow it to wear off and see how your body responds. You can decide whether the procedure is worth repeating, or if your symptoms are under control without it. The goal is to determine which treatments you need to maintain your improvements; you're searching for the best symptom reduction with the fewest side effects.

Pelvic Floor Physical Therapy: Regular Checkups

By the time you reach this final stage in your IC journey, you should be ready to graduate from weekly physical therapy. You'll be an expert in your own pelvic floor, and can self-identify any dysfunction that reemerges. Many patients continue with monthly or quarterly maintenance visits to make sure they're not missing anything, but you should be able to decrease the frequency of visits by this point.

Your pelvic floor physical therapist should guide your flare management program and help identify which self-care treatments are most beneficial for you. Specific symptoms are often associated with tension or dysfunction in a particular location. With your PT's help, you will recognize which home treatments will provide the most benefit. For example, bladder symptoms are often associated with tight muscles in the pelvic floor near the urethra, so an increase in those symptoms should prompt either self-release of a specific internal trigger point or a visit to your physical therapist for additional help. Hip pain is often associated with tight muscles in the pelvic floor and surrounding areas, so additional stretching may be your best source of relief. Since you identified the root causes of your specific symptoms in Stage II, you'll now be able to address them quickly when they arise.

Self-Care: Healthy Habits

By now your optimal self-care program should be a daily habit. Daily stretching, fascial release, and trigger point work should remain a part of your program. Patients who have successfully cleared their internal pelvic floor dysfunction still do a quick check at least once a week to release any new internal trigger points. Continue to stretch and make sure inflammation doesn't build in the fascia to prevent problems from cropping up again. This is vital to managing your condition and preventing symptoms from recurring.

You can expand your exercise program, as well. Consider activities that support, rather than hinder, your pelvic health. For instance, yoga, swimming, walking, or a modified Pilates program can give you cardiovascular exercise while loosening tight pelvic muscles.

Diet: Be Confident in Your Choices

All trigger foods should have been identified and eliminated by now. The challenge is adding foods back into your diet to compensate for the items you removed. Your goal is to make a healthy, satisfying diet second nature. Maybe you can occasionally sneak a taste of a favorite food you know you shouldn't have, or go out to dinner with family confident you can manage the consequences. Continue to try new recipes, and work to ensure you eat a healthy, balanced diet.

Complementary and Alternative Medicine: Keep What Helps

If you have already identified a program of vitamins, supplements, and alternative therapies that are beneficial, then continue with your regimen. Experiment with other options, though, and be on the lookout for new products that come onto the market.

Mental Health: Believe in Yourself

Improving your mental and emotional health should also be a habit at this stage. Whether you've found daily meditation, weekly therapy, yoga classes, or another technique to be most beneficial, make sure it's a stable part of your routine.

You should also start to feel a sense of control over your condition. After all, you have all the knowledge necessary to understand what's going on inside your body. You shouldn't feel anxious about your condition. Instead, you should feel confident that you know what to expect and can handle any problems that arise.

This may be a great time to start giving back to your IC community. Consider founding or participating in an IC support group, or volunteering if there's another charitable organization you feel passionate about. Or, take a few minutes each day to spread hope in the IC community online, encouraging others going through a tough time.

IC Flares: Your Flare-Busting Plan

Successfully managing an IC flare is all about having a plan. You've spent months or years finding out how to manage your IC; now you just need to apply that hard-won knowledge to your flare. Sometimes the pain or symptoms of a flare can be scary or disorienting, so a detailed, written plan for addressing them is important to have. Many of my patients will print out the following form and put it on their fridge or bulletin board so they're prepared for a sudden flare.

Creating a personal flare-busting plan is simple. First, write down the three things you do by yourself that relieve your symptoms. The only rule is they have to be in your direct control, and don't require help from anyone else.

PERSONAL FLARE-BUSTING PLAN

Three things I can do myself to decrease my symptoms:

1. _____

2. _____

3. _____

Most effective medical treatment to help me during this time (circle one):

Physical therapy

Acupuncture

Bladder instillations

Neuromodulation

Massage therapy

Break-through pain medication

Other: _____

My IC comfort foods:

1. _____

2. _____

3. _____

4. _____

5. _____

Contributing factors to this flare (circle all that apply):

Prolonged sitting

New/increased physical activity

Change in diet

Change in medications

New procedure

Stress

Stopped self-care regimen

Sexual activity

Other: _____

Examples of Things to Do Yourself

- Deep breathing
- Medications
- Meditating
- Skin rolling
- Stretching
- Trigger point release
- Warm bath
- Yoga
- Calling a friend
- Attend an IC support group meeting

During the course of your recovery, you'll have noticed which medical treatments show benefit the fastest. Common examples include physical therapy, acupuncture, bladder instillations, or breakthrough pain medication. Focus on the treatment that gives you the best, most immediate results. When you feel a flare building, get an appointment as quickly as possible.

The next part of your plan is your IC comfort foods. This section is particularly important if you're highly diet sensitive. The foods and drinks on this list should be meals you love to eat and that you are fully confident contain no triggers.

Finally, take control over the cause of your flare. The last section of your plan asks what prompted the problem. If you look objectively at your past week, it's likely a reason will emerge. Sometimes the reason is clear and obvious, but other times it's more subtle. For instance, emotional stress may play a role, even if you're not consciously aware that something is bothering you. Identify all factors you believe contributed to your flare: This will help you demystify the process and retake control of your health. Be confident that a flare is just a flare—nothing more. It doesn't mean you have to start your journey over again. The flare, even if it's a difficult one, is happening to a different, more prepared body. You have power over your flares.

CHARTING YOUR RECOVERY

	Stage I: Manage Your Symptoms	Stage II: Address Underlying Issues	Stage III: Living Successfully with IC	✓
Oral medication	Start medication, observe benefits, and side effects	Fine-tune medications to increase benefits and reduce side effects	Find your permanent regimen; reduce or eliminate unnecessary medication	
Bladder treatments	Try bladder instillations	If bladder instillations are not effective, try neurostimulation or behavioral training	Determine whether bladder treatments are an integral part of your ongoing treatment, or just for flare management	
Pelvic floor PT	Try pelvic floor PT and determine how much your pelvic floor contributes to your pain	Continue with pelvic floor PT; work on the "why"—figure out underlying causes and work to address them	Identify the root cause of each of your symptoms, and be confident in addressing them yourself.	
Self-care	Begin daily stretching regimen; work on fascial and trigger point release	Tailor stretching and strengthening to your specific problem areas; become comfortable with internal and external trigger point release at home	Make your self-care program a habit, and be confident in your techniques when you experience a flare.	
Diet	Eliminate the most common problem foods with IC; determine level of your food sensitivity	Take the next step with your diet: add foods back in or find additional trigger foods to remove	Find a diet that you are happy and comfortable with; continue exploring new recipes and ingredients	
Complementary treatments	Try something new	Add something to your daily regimen	Find the alternative treatment most effective for your case.	
Mental health	Work to relieve stress and relax the nervous system; practice deep breathing; identify underlying sources of emotional distress	Actively work on your mental health: consider meditation, cognitive behavioral therapy, a psychologist, or an interstitial cystitis support group	Feel a sense of control over your physical health and condition; give back to others	
Goals	Take action; see a change in your condition, and learn what your IC responds best to	Develop specific recovery goals; keep going, and stay positive through bumps in the road	Successfully manage flares when they arise; be proud of how far you've come; regain your life!	

Takeaways

- **Manage your condition and know your body.** By now you've acquired a wealth of hard-won knowledge about your body. Focus on the treatments that work for you, and refine your daily program to deliver the most benefits. Listen to your body: There will be times when you need additional treatment, and times when the path is smooth and easy.

- **Have a plan for flares.** With your day-to-day symptoms under control, your biggest challenge will be dealing with the occasional flare. With a detailed flare management plan in place, your response will be rapid and effective. Written steps are vital for this process. Be confident and trust that the same methods that brought you this far on your IC journey will see you through the occasional flare, as well.

- **Live your life!** This is the time to gradually regain your normal life. Add activities back into your schedule, or replace things you used to do with new interests that are better for your body. You will always have IC, but it doesn't have to define you. Thousands of people live healthy, happy lives with interstitial cystitis. Make sure you're one of them!

For New and Veteran Patients

For new patients, don't get complacent at this stage. This can be an exciting time as you get to regain parts of your life that had been put on hold because of IC, but don't neglect the healthy habits you built to get here.

Also remember that if a flare happens—and they do—that it doesn't ever mean that you're back to square one. Your body has a new normal now, and your job is to get your body back to that level as quickly as you can after a flare. You have the tools, and know what works. Be confident!

For veteran patients, this can be a time where you gain a new perspective and acceptance of where you are in life, and how your journey has shaped you. Hopefully dealing with your IC will feel less like a battle with each passing day. Find new activities to replace anything you've had to give up, and think about how far you've come. You'll also need to fight complacency, but you've worked hard to get here, so be proud of your achievements.

APPENDIX:

PRACTICAL IC SOLUTIONS

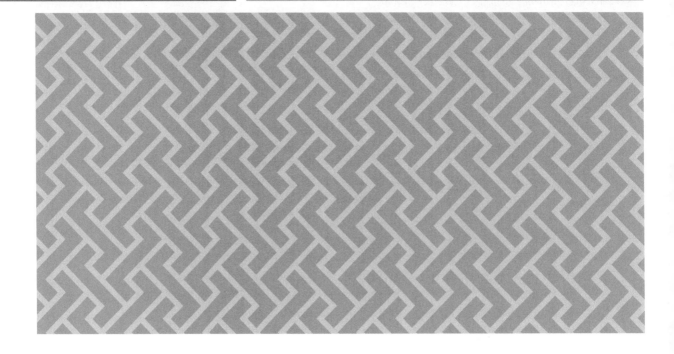

How to Assemble Your Medical Team

Whether you're newly diagnosed or have battled the condition for years, choose your medical team carefully. Dealing with IC requires a multi-disciplinary approach. At a minimum, you'll need to find a urologist or urogynecologist who specializes in pelvic pain conditions, a pelvic floor physical therapist, and a pain-management doctor. Many patients also benefit from a professional to help with the psychological challenges of IC.

The most important thing is to find medical practitioners who *want* to treat patients like you. Most doctors aren't accustomed to the kind of care it takes to treat chronic conditions, such as IC. There won't be a quick fix or an easy answer, and you'll be working together for a long time. When you find a specialist in the area, you'll know she has dedicated her professional career to patients like you. Here are the specialists you need to find:

- **Urologist or urogynecologist:** This is the primary doctor who will guide your care. She will prescribe the majority, if not all, of your medications, including pain medications, other oral medications, or muscle relaxants that can ease tension in your pelvic floor in conjunction with stretching and physical therapy. If you receive weekly bladder instillations, they'll be conducted by this doctor. When you're trying to find oral medications that work for you and to fine-tune their dosage, your doctor will probably want to see you every four to six weeks. Also, she will usually be responsible for trigger point injections, nerve blocks, BOTOX treatments, and other procedures. Find a doctor who's familiar with IC patients and with these procedures—preferably one who has made pelvic health a specialty.

- **Pelvic floor physical therapist:** It's likely your physical therapist will be the practitioner you see most often, usually once or twice a week. She (pelvic floor physical therapists are almost exclusively women) will take time to help you understand the condition and the anatomy of your pelvic floor. Her hands-on treatment will focus on loosening the tight muscles and fascia around your pelvic floor, both externally and internally. She'll guide your self-care methods, including stretching and exercises to strengthen your pelvic floor and core. She will evaluate your posture, teach you about behavioral therapy, and provide other practical suggestions for pelvic health. Also, your physical therapist will probably have recommendations for doctors who provide excellent care for IC patients.

- **Mental and emotional health practitioners:** There are many types of practitioners who work with mental and emotional health, and patients can benefit greatly from finding a specialist with whom they're comfortable—such as a psychologist, sex therapist, cognitive-behavioral therapist, or meditation teacher, to name a few. This doesn't have to be a weekly appointment; even a single visit can be extremely helpful in learning strategies for dealing with the stress and challenges that often accompany an IC diagnosis.

- **Pain-management specialist:** If you have high levels of uncontrolled pain, add this specialist to your team. Your pain-management doctor focuses on treating and managing chronic pain, and may also administer nerve blocks within the pelvic floor, low back, or sacrum to calm the nerves of the pelvis and reduce symptoms. You'll probably visit this specialist every four to six weeks early in your treatment, when you're trying to find the right drug or combination of drugs to deal with your pain. As you settle into a treatment program that works for you, these visits should decrease, and should eventually become unnecessary.

"An expert can put together a treatment plan that your local doctor or physical therapist can follow, combining the knowledge of a specialist with the convenience of a local practitioner."

What If I Don't Have a Local Specialist?

Unfortunately, there are relatively few experts in pelvic pain in the United States, and not everyone has local access to a true specialist. Both doctors and physical therapists that focus on the pelvic floor and chronic pelvic pain are rare, and may not be located close enough to make regular visits a possibility.

So consider travelling—at least to get an initial opinion from a true specialist in the field. It can ensure a correct diagnosis, giving you certainty about the condition. And an expert can put together a treatment plan that your local doctor or physical therapist can follow, combining the knowledge of a specialist with the convenience of a local practitioner.

Two primary obstacles arise when patients consider travelling for better medical care: cost and the difficulties of travelling with IC. When it comes to cost, it's important to look at the big picture. IC can be an expensive condition, with different medications, doctor visits, physical therapy, and other assorted medical costs. But the goal of every good medical practitioner should be to help you become self-sufficient in your own treatment as soon as possible. Some patients spend years being treated by a local doctor or physical therapist with no detailed knowledge about the condition—so if visiting a specialist puts you on the path to healing, you'll actually save money.

The other hurdle to overcome is the difficulty of travelling with interstitial cystitis. This can be a major challenge, depending on the severity of your symptoms. Prolonged sitting in an airplane or car can exacerbate symptoms, and worrying about finding a bathroom when the urge strikes can cause anxiety. Yes, the change to your routine and the stress associated with travel can cause a flare—but it's worth it in this instance.

You deserve the best medical care and advice you can find. Without it, you may spend months or years wondering whether you really even have IC! By visiting an acknowledged expert in the field, you'll get answers that are invaluable to your IC journey. Plus, a specialist can create a treatment regimen that your local practitioner can follow. Many experts offer phone consultations after your initial visit, allowing you to check in with a specialist without even leaving your house. Dealing with IC is a lifelong journey, and it's certainly worth ensuring you get the best possible care and advice from the beginning.

Make the Most of Your Doctor's Appointment

To expand the list first presented in chapter 4 (page 48), here's a bit more detail on what you should bring to your appointment to make the most of your limited time with your doctor—and to ensure your concerns are heard.

Written list of your worst 3 to 4 symptoms

- Make sure you've thought these through and have written them all down. Present them in the order of severity.

Other symptoms that may or may not be related

- If you have other symptoms that might (or might not) be related, make a separate list of them. You don't want to give your doctor a list of twelve different symptoms and ask her to come up with a condition that explains them all. It's important to differentiate between your primary symptoms and ones that may or may not be caused by your condition.

Symptom diary

- A detailed symptom diary (see chapter 2) can provide helpful information to your doctor. It also presents your symptoms in a way that's easy for your doctor to visualize.

Bladder diary

- A detailed bladder diary can provide specific information about your urinary habits and give objective information to your doctor. By having completed a bladder diary before your doctor's appointment, you can save yourself several weeks and another visit. It's much more convincing to hand your doctor a log of the number of times you went to the bathroom over the previous days than to just tell her, "I have to go all the time." Keep this diary for at least three days prior to your appointment (see chapter 4).

Written timeline of symptoms/treatments

- This can give the doctor a more complete picture of your symptoms and what has been done to address them. For example, knowing you took two rounds of antibiotics, and what type, for a potential UTI a few months ago can help your doctor rule out a UTI and consider IC instead.

Any previous testing results

- Similarly, you should bring in any test results you have. Whenever you leave a doctor's office, get a copy of your test results and take them with you to future appointments.

Easing/aggravating factors

- If you've noticed a correlation between your symptoms and other factors in your life—such as specific foods, activities, stress levels, or exercise—report these to your doctor.

Medications you've tried or are currently taking

- Your doctor will want to know what medications you've tried to treat your symptoms, and whether you're currently on any medications. You should also write the most important ones down, including dosage levels, so your doctor can know what has and hasn't worked for you.

Travelling with Interstitial Cystitis

Let's face it, travelling with IC is hard. Urinary symptoms can make travel a challenge, and trips often involve a lot of time sitting, which can flare symptoms. Here are a few tips for making travel less scary, and for restoring your confidence en route.

- If you travel by car, plan restroom stops along your route. Make sure your travelling companions are aware of the plan before you begin, and don't feel embarrassed about these scheduled stops. Most people are grateful for the opportunity to get out of the car and stretch their legs.

- A long drive can be difficult because you are seated, which can exacerbate pelvic floor dysfunction. A seat cushion designed to relieve pressure on the pelvic floor can make driving a more pleasant experience.

- When you get out of the car for a regular stop, stretch your legs and pelvis for a few minutes before resuming your journey. Especially stretch the muscles shortened with sitting— the hamstrings and hip flexors in particular. And don't forget the pelvic floor squat stretch.

- If you travel by plane, bring your own seat cushion and try to get an aisle seat. If you are concerned about your urinary symptoms, let a flight attendant know before you take off. You can also bring a short letter from your doctor or PT explaining your condition, which can help ensure you get an aisle seat and any additional help you might need. Take a look at the example on the opposite page.

When you travel, realize you're going to place additional strain on your body, so you may have to deal with increased symptoms over the next several days. Following the tips described previously can reduce the toll that travel takes on your body— but still, consider scheduling an "easy" day or two after each leg of your trip. Acknowledge that you may not be able to have a full day of activities after a long travel day, and give yourself permission to take some time off when you reach your destination. It's a good idea to focus on stretching and self-care after a journey, and, if a hot bath is available, it can be a welcome relaxation at the end of a day of travel. Have your written flare-busting plan (chapter 15) ready for use after travel.

PATIENT RESOURCE TRAVEL LETTER

To Whom It May Concern:

_____ has a bladder pain condition called interstitial cystitis.
It can cause the frequent and sometimes urgent need to urinate. This condition is very painful and many equate it to
the feeling of glass shards in the bladder or the worst UTI imaginable. Sitting for long periods of time is also painful
and difficult. You can assist with the travel challenges associated with the condition in the following ways:

1. Allow for _____ to sit in an aisle seat, preferably close to a restroom.

2. Allow for _____ to get up and stand for short periods of time.

3. Be compassionate about the difficulties travel imposes for _____ ,
   even though there may be no outward signs of the condition.

Thank you for your understanding.

_____
(Signed by you, your doctor, or physical therapist)

"After you've applied heat, your muscles will be more elastic, so now is a good time to stretch."

IC-Friendly Meal Plans

One thing many patients find helpful when changing their diet for IC is to create a meal plan for each week. This is also a great way to involve your family or significant other in your IC journey: Take the opportunity to educate them about your condition and how they can help. As you learn about your trigger foods, this will soon become second nature—but, in the early stages, having a plan can make all the difference.

Ice or Heat for Interstitial Cystitis?

Many patients wonder whether they should apply ice or heat to their pelvic and abdominal regions to relieve IC symptoms. Ice is typically used to prevent an acute inflammatory response after an injury, while heat loosens muscles and releases tension. There are both ice packs and heating pads shaped for use in the pelvic and groin area.

If you've had a specific incident that may be causing inflammation and pain—such as sitting for a long period of time, having sexual intercourse, or suffering another acute injury—ice can be useful. Wrap it in a pillowcase until it's tolerable and not too cold. Don't ice a particular area for more than fifteen minutes at a time, and wait at least an hour before icing again.

On the other hand, many patients find their muscles loosen with heat. It's one reason a warm bath is a favorite home remedy for symptoms. Applying moist heat can also create a sensation of warmth and relaxation in the area, which can help decrease symptoms. You can leave a heat source in place for longer than ice: about thirty minutes. After you've applied the heat, your muscles will be more elastic, so now is a good time to stretch, as well.

In general, more IC patients seem to be helped by heat than by ice. A warm bath, hot tub, or heating pad can be very beneficial. In conjunction with stretching, heat can help relax and loosen the muscles surrounding the pelvic area. However, as with all treatments, let your body be your guide. If ice helps, don't be afraid to keep using it. Experiment with both, and find what works best for you.

Sitting and Interstitial Cystitis

We know the seated position puts a lot of strain on the pelvic floor, which is already tight and irritated with IC. Prolonged sitting is one of the worst things an IC patient can do, exacerbating symptoms and flaring pelvic floor dysfunction. Though it's impossible to eliminate sitting completely, there are several things you can do to make it less stressful on your pelvic floor:

- Reduce prolonged periods of sitting. If you do need to be seated, stand up and move around at least once an hour to loosen your pelvic floor. Even giving yourself a few minutes' break from sitting can be helpful.

- Work to make your seated position more comfortable for your pelvic floor. Many seat cushions effectively reduce the strain of sitting on the pelvis. Different versions work well for different patients, so try a few options before purchasing one. Many manufacturers have a return policy for this reason, so try a cushion for a week or so before making a final decision. Take your seat cushion with you when you drive; use it at work; and make your favorite chair at home substantially more relaxing for your pelvic floor.

- Have your physical therapist examine your sitting posture and make any necessary adjustments. Even a small change can make a big difference. You can bring photos of yourself sitting in common areas around the house (couch, lounge, dinner table, etc.), and have your PT troubleshoot those locations with you. This is important, even if you don't notice your pain being directly related to sitting. Even with no apparent connection, the stress sitting places on the pelvic floor can be a contributing factor to other symptoms.

Exercising with Interstitial Cystitis

Exercise is an important component of overall health, and needs to be part of your daily routine. However, certain activities can place additional stress on the pelvic floor and should be avoided. As always, when you start an exercise routine, build gradually toward your goal.

Walking on a flat surface is always a good place to start. This loosens the muscles surrounding the pelvic floor. Going uphill or downhill can strain leg muscles. Running is much more vigorous and can jar the pelvic floor. If you were a runner before receiving your diagnosis, it might take some time before you're able to run without exacerbating your symptoms, but it's a good goal to work toward. If you weren't a dedicated runner, it's best to choose a form of exercise that doesn't place as much strain on the body.

Swimming is a great exercise for interstitial cystitis patients. It loosens the legs, promotes flexibility, and is a great full-body workout. When you swim, you work against the resistance of the water, and you won't jostle your pelvic floor as you might with running or vigorous walking. If you're starting off slowly with exercise, or if you find exercise tends to flare your symptoms, walking in a pool can be great. And, if you have back, knee, or hip pain, exercising in water can be a lifesaver. Many gyms or cities have a heated pool for community use. Some patients even use a hot tub for exercise, walking in place in the water. Stretching in a pool or hot tub can also be easier on the body and can relax the muscles.

Yoga is another option with many benefits. It can increase flexibility, improve strength, and be a form of meditation and stress relief. If you're new to yoga, begin with a restorative yoga class and gradually work your way into more challenging programs.

Some exercises aren't recommended for IC patients. Biking, for instance, puts a great deal of strain on the pelvic floor—even in people without IC! —and forces you to sit for a long period of time. Plus, the horn of the bike seat directly compresses part of the pudendal nerve and pelvic floor muscles. Also, when you're starting out, avoid strength workouts on the muscles that connect with the pelvis. Abdominal crunches and inner thigh and hamstring exercises can have a ripple effect throughout the pelvic region. Exercise these muscle groups by walking, swimming, or doing yoga instead. Many patients also report that working out on an elliptical machine tends to flare symptoms—perhaps because of the unusual pattern of motion. If you long to resume biking or using an elliptical, consider trying a short session after you're symptom-free for a while to determine whether a small amount of the exercise will flare your symptoms. Your pelvic floor physical therapist can give you personalized advice on your exercise program.

Whatever type of exercise you choose, try to do it each day, in a way that raises your heart rate and challenges your body without flaring your symptoms. Be patient as you work your way into your exercise routine, and allow your body to become accustomed to the additional exertion. Exercise is an important part of your healing journey: Keep that in mind and choose something you enjoy doing.

Work and Interstitial Cystitis

Working with IC can be challenging. Many jobs typically require prolonged sitting at a workstation. Urinary symptoms can make it difficult to sit through long meetings, or can make you feel like you're constantly heading to the bathroom. Once you're on the road to recovery, you need to optimize your work environment for your condition.

The first thing to do is minimize the amount of time you spend sitting. Stand up when you're talking on the phone or read while leaning over your desk and stretching your hamstrings. If you're seated, make sure to stand up and move around at least every forty-five minutes (or earlier, if you start feeling symptoms increasing). There are adjustable sit-to-stand desks that allow you to work while standing or you can install additions that rest on top of your desk to reach standing height.

Some patients bring in a simple description of their condition, including what their employer can do to help. Many employers are sympathetic and accommodating. If you're hesitant about sharing the nature of the condition, just let people know you are struggling with "low back pain." Most people have experienced that at some point in their lives, and it can explain why you're unable to sit for long periods of time.

The most important thing about working with interstitial cystitis is being confident enough to do what you need to do to stay healthy. Yes, you may need to call a break or slip out during a meeting to use the bathroom, but most of the time the people you're meeting with will be glad of a quick break themselves.

Socializing with Interstitial Cystitis

IC can be isolating—at a time when friendship can be crucially important. So be honest with your support system! If you go out to eat, suggest sitting at one of the higher bar tables where you can stand rather than sit. The "low back pain" excuse can be effective here, as well, if you aren't comfortable sharing the nature of IC with your friends. Look at the restaurant's menu online before you go so you'll have time to think about which options are best for your diet. You can also change how you socialize with people. Invite friends to go for a short walk or attend a yoga class together. Or, if going out isn't an option, invite someone over to your home, even if it's only for a little while. Video chatting can be a surrogate for in-person socializing if you're unable to meet in person.

It may take courage, but, if you share about your condition, your close friends will be eager to help. This can be a great source of comfort during difficult times, so don't let IC force you to keep your friends at arm's length.

Sex and Interstitial Cystitis

The majority of IC patients have some form of pain with sex, typically stemming from the pelvic floor dysfunction that accompanies the condition. This can be frustrating and can put a strain on relationships, but there are several things you can do to regain a healthy sex life.

In women, sexual pain either accompanies entry or is deep vaginal pain with intercourse—both can be present at the same time and are due to pelvic floor dysfunction. Pain with entry is more typical for IC patients, because it takes place near the muscles that control the urethra. Intercourse can prompt pain, urgency, or urethral burning. Even if you don't have immediate pain with intercourse, note whether you experience an increase in symptoms after sex: for some patients, the flared symptoms can linger for days.

Although we often think of painful sex as a problem that affects women, men experience pain with sex, as well. Sexual pain with men manifests as pain with erection, pain following ejaculation, and lingering symptoms after sex. Maintaining an erection and ejaculating both involve a contraction of the pelvic floor, which may already be irritated due to IC. Stretching and self-care prior to sex can help mitigate the strain of sexual activity. Men often experience a feeling of urinary urgency after sex, which can be paired with a hesitant flow of urine as the pelvic floor struggles to relax.

Pain with sex can take an emotional toll on relationships, and the fear of pain in connection with such an intimate event can be difficult to overcome. If you struggle with this, consider seeing a sex therapist. These specialists focus on intimacy issues between couples and work to foster a healthy dialogue about the problem and ways to express intimacy other than with intercourse.

There are physical steps you can take to mitigate pain with sex, too. For women, a vaginal dilator can be useful. It can help you overcome the fear of pain with intercourse in a setting where you're in complete control, letting you get used to the feeling of penetration without pain. These dilators come in several sizes, so you can get comfortable with a small size before proceeding to a larger one. Consult your pelvic floor physical therapist about how to use it.

Before having sex, go through your pelvic floor stretching routine (see chapter 10), which can relax the pelvic floor and surrounding muscles. Relieving internal trigger points prior to intercourse either manually or with the crystal wand can reduce pain with entry or during intercourse. Use plenty of personal lubricant to minimize discomfort during entry.

It's important you are comfortable and able to relax during sex. The muscles of your legs and inner thighs should not be tensed: For women, the happy baby position—lying on your back with your knees brought toward your chest—automatically relaxes the pelvic floor and may be a good option. You can also try lying on your side with your partner behind you: Many patients find this position comfortable because it allows the legs to relax. Deep, diaphragmatic breathing during initial penetration and any other periods of discomfort can also help loosen the pelvic floor. And good communication is essential. Trust that your partner will modify the movement—or stop completely—if necessary.

Both men and women with IC may want to stretch after sex. Your pelvic floor will naturally tighten during intercourse, and stretching it out afterward keeps trigger points from forming. If any areas feel painful or inflamed after intercourse, now might be a good time to ice them. Remember to wrap the ice in a piece of cloth, such as a pillowcase, and never ice a single area for more than fifteen minutes at a time.

The toll painful sex takes on relationships is often a hidden cost of interstitial cystitis. But you can minimize the toll. Above all, be honest with your partner. In the early days of your treatment, your pelvic floor may not be able to tolerate intercourse: Instead, work to find other ways to express your love and intimacy. When you are ready for intercourse, make sure you're communicating freely with your partner, and know that you're able to stop if you begin to experience pain or symptoms. With treatment, pelvic floor physical therapy, and self-care techniques, it is certainly possible to rediscover a healthy sex life.

Managing IC on a Budget

IC can be expensive, and you may start to see the financial burden of the condition. On bad days, resist the urge to throw up your hands and decide you're spending money for nothing. Remember: Treating your IC is an investment in your future. Don't put short-term considerations ahead of long-term goals. If you try to save money by not getting treatment, there will be a long-term cost. Your symptoms may worsen until you can't work, or they may end up taking much longer to treat than if you'd gotten help early. There are many ways to see meaningful, sustained improvement without breaking the bank. Here are a few.

Specialists Are Worth the Extra Money

This can be a difficult choice: Should you just see your primary care doctor, or should you find a specialist who may be more expensive, or require a longer trip to visit? For most patients with IC, the specialist is worth the extra cost and inconvenience. Remember that she works with patients like you on a daily basis. Yes, a specialist may be more expensive for a single appointment, but if it speeds your recovery the visit may result in significant savings over time. Even seeing a specialist just a few times can put you on the right track. If you don't have a local specialist, many clinics have specific out-of-town programs that help you make the most of your visit.

Ask About Generic or Over-the-Counter Drugs

Often, when it comes to medication, a doctor's first thought is to prescribe a brand-name drug that's new to the market, but a large number of medications for IC have generic versions. Certain medications may also be available in less powerful doses as over-the-counter drugs, which do not require a prescription. Always have a conversation with your doctor about your medication, and don't be afraid to ask whether there's a lower-cost or generic option available. There are online resources that compare the cost of a prescription drug at different pharmacies, so you can shop around for the best price, too.

For drugs without a generic version, consider contacting the manufacturer directly. Some drug or medical device companies have patient assistance programs, to which they donate money to help patients get the treatment they need.

Take Your Health into Your Own Hands

Self-care is among the most important aspects of managing IC. Patients who put in the most work see the best results. And most of these techniques—both physical and mental—are free! If you have to forego some treatment options because of cost, make sure you invest time in taking care of yourself. Stretching, self-massage, deep breathing, warm baths, meditation, and many more self-care techniques can have major benefits—and you don't need a doctor to administer the treatment.

Do Bladder Instillations Yourself

Many patients who are helped by bladder instillations ask their doctor to teach them how to self-catheterize and do the procedure at home. That way, you can pick up your prescription at the pharmacy and avoid the expense of the office visit. This is also helpful when travelling, or for immediate flare management.

Turn Yourself (or Your Partner) into Your Physical Therapist

Your physical therapist will be happy to teach you self-care techniques. Learn from her, and have her teach your partner, as well. You can decrease the frequency of physical therapy appointments by doing more work yourself. While you should still make sure you see your PT regularly to assess your progress and guide your self-care, this approach can help you see better results with fewer visits.

Focus on What Really Helps

Spend some extra time and money early in your IC journey to learn what's most helpful for your particular condition. Everyone is different, so a systematic approach will let you know which treatments will have the most benefit for you. That way, you can then focus only on the most helpful therapies, and be confident you're investing time and money wisely.

RESOURCES FOR IC

Here are some helpful resources for more information on interstitial cystitis.

The Interstitial Cystitis Association (ICA):
The leading IC patient advocacy group, the ICA has excellent information about interstitial cystitis, listings of local support groups, and other resources for patients. www.ichelp.org

American Urological Association (AUA) IC Guidelines: Updated in 2014, the AUA IC Guidelines provide a summary of clinical trials in IC and recommend six different lines of treatment to be tried by patients. www.auanet.org/education/guidelines/ic-bladder-pain-syndrome.cfm

IC Network: The IC Network has information for patients, a large patient forum, and a store where common IC supplements, books, and other items are sold. www.ic-network.org

American Physical Therapy Association (APTA):
The APTA section on women's health has patient information, as well as a listing of the board-certified physical therapists (Women's Clinical Specialists, or WCS) that can help you locate an experienced PT who can treat both men and women. www.apta.org

International Pelvic Pain Society (IPPS): The IPPS is a multidisciplinary society that focuses on pelvic pain conditions. Here you can find a list of medical practitioners who have registered in specializing in conditions such as interstitial cystitis. www.pelvicpain.org

American Urogynecological Society (AUGS): The AUGS website has a "find a provider" link to help you find a urogynecologist who can help treat IC in your area. It also has a blog with patient information and resources for all kinds of pelvic floor dysfunction. www.voicesforpfd.org

PelvicSanity: This information website, founded by Nicole Cozean, offers practical positive advice for patients with interstitial cystitis and pelvic floor dysfunction. Here you can download the resources mentioned in this book, including worksheets, images, and checklists. www.PelvicSanity.com

MAIN REFERENCES

Al-Zahrani, A., and J. Gajewski. "Long-Term Efficacy and Tolerability of Pentosan Polysuphate Sodium in the Treatment of Bladder Pain Syndrome." *Canadian Urological Association Journal* 5, no. 2 (April 2011): 113–18.

Berry, S., M. Elliott, M. Suttorp, et al. "Prevalence of Symptoms of Bladder Pain Syndrome/Interstitial Cystitis Among Adult Females in the United States." *The Journal of Urology* 186, no. 2 (August 2011): 540–44.

Clemens, J., M. Elliott, M. Suttorp, and S. Berry. "Temporal Ordering of Interstitial Cystitis/Bladder Pain Syndrome and Non-Bladder Conditions." *Urology* 80, no. 6 (December 2012): 1227–31.

Dimitrakov, J., K. Kroenke, W. Steers, et al. "Pharmacological Management of Painful Bladder Syndrome/Interstitial Cystitis: A Systematic Review." *Archives of Internal Medicine* 167, no. 18 (October 2007): 1922–29.

FitzGerald, M., R. Anderson, J. Potts, et al. "Randomized Multicenter Feasibility Trial of Myofascial Physical Therapy for Treatment of Urologic Chronic Pelvic Pain Syndrome." *The Journal of Urology* 182, no. 2 (June 2009): 570–80.

FitzGerald, M., C. Payne, E. Lukacz, et al. "Randomized Multicenter Clinical Trial of Myofascial Physical Therapy in Women with Interstitial Cystitis/Painful Bladder Syndrome (IC/PBS) and Pelvic Floor Tenderness." *The Journal of Urology* 187, no. 6 (June 2012): 2113–18.

FitzGerald, M., and R. Kotarinos. "Rehabilitation of the Short Pelvic Floor. I: Background and Patient Evaluation. *International Urogynecology Journal* 14, no. 4 (October 2003): 261–68.

FitzGerald, M., and R. Kotarinos. "Rehabilitation of the Short Pelvic Floor. II: Treatment of the Patient with the Short Pelvic Floor. *International Urogynecology Journal* 14, no. 4 (October 2003): 269–75.

Forrest, J., J. Nickel, and R. Moldwin. "Chronic Prostatitis/Chronic Pelvic Pain Syndrome and Male Interstitial Cystitis: Enigmas and Opportunities." *Urology* 69, no. 4 Supplement (April 2007): 60–63.

Friedlander, J., B. Shorter, and R. Moldwin. "Diet and its Role in Interstitial Cystitis/Bladder Pain Syndrome (IC/BPS) and Comorbid Conditions." *BJU International* 109, no. 11 (June 2012): 1584–91.

Goldstein, A., C. Pukall, and I. Goldstein. *When Sex Hurts: A Woman's Guide to Banishing Sexual Pain*. Cambridge, MA: Da Capo Lifelong Books, 2011.

Hanno, P., D. Burks, J. Clemens, et al. "AUA Guidelines for the Diagnosis and Treatment of Interstitial Cystitis/Bladder Pain Syndrome." *The Journal of Urology* 185, no. 6 (June 2011): 2162–70.

Hepner, K., K. Watkins, M. Elliott, et al. "Suicidal Ideation among Patients with Bladder Pain Syndrome/Interstitial Cystitis." *Urology* 80, no. 2 (August 2012): 280–85.

Masheb, R., R. Kerns, C. Lozano, et al. "A Randomized Clinical Trial for Women with Vulvodynia: Cognitive-Behavioral Therapy vs. Supportive Psychotherapy." *Pain* 141, nos. 1–2 (January 2009): 31–40.

Meijlink, J. "Interstitial Cystitis and the Painful Bladder: A Brief History of Nomenclature, Definitions, and Criteria." *International Journal of Urology* 21, Issue Supplement S1 (April 2014): 4–12.

Moldwin, R. *The Interstitial Cystitis Survival Guide: Your Guide to the Latest Treatment Options and Coping Strategies.* Oakland, CA: New Harbinger Publications, 2000.

O'Leary, M. P., G. R. Sant, F. J. Fowler Jr., et al. "The Interstitial Cystitis Symptom Index and Problem Index." *Urology* 49, no. 5 Supplement 1 (May 1997): 58–63.

Oyama, I. A., A. Rejba, J. C. Lukban, et al. "Modified Thiele Massage as Therapeutic Intervention for Female Patients with Interstitial Cystitis and High-Tone Pelvic Floor Dysfunction." *Urology* 64, no. 5 (November 2004): 862–65.

Parsons, C., and V. Tatsis. "Prevalence of Interstitial Cystitis in Young Women." *Urology* 64, no. 5 (November 2004): 866–70.

Stein, A. *Heal Pelvic Pain: The Proven Stretching, Strengthening, and Nutrition Program for Relieving Pain, Incontinence, I.B.S., and Other Symptoms without Surgery.* New York: McGraw-Hill Education, 2008.

Suskind, A., S. Berry, B. Ewing, et al. "The Prevalence and Overlap of Interstitial Cystitis/Bladder Pain Syndrome and Chronic Prostatitis/Chronic Pelvic Pain Syndrome in Men; Results of the RAND Interstitial Cystitis Epidemiology (RICE) Male Study." *The Journal of Urology* 189, no. 1 (January 2013): 141–45.

Vickers, A. J., A. M. Cronin, A. C. Maschino, et al. "Acupuncture for Chronic Pain: Individual Patient Data Meta-Analysis." *Archives of Internal Medicine* 172, no. 19 (October 2012): 1444–53.

Watkins, K., N. Eberhart, L. Hilton, et al. "Depressive Disorders and Panic Attacks in Women with Bladder Pain Syndrome/Interstitial Cystitis: A Population-Based Study." *General Hospital Psychiatry* 33, no. 2 (March–April 2011): 143–49.

Weiss, J. M. "Pelvic Floor Myofascial Trigger Points: Manual Therapy for Interstitial Cystitis and the Urgency-Frequency Syndrome." *The Journal of Urology* 166, no. 6 (December 2001): 2226–31.

Zeidan, F., J. Grant, C. Brown, et al. "Mindfulness Meditation-Related Pain Relief: Evidence for Unique Brain Mechanisms in the Regulation of Pain." *Neuroscience Letters* 520, no. 2 (June 2012):165–73.

ACKNOWLEDGMENTS

With deep gratitude we would like to acknowledge some of the people who helped bring this book into being. Our first thanks go to our agent, Anne Marie O'Farrell, for her initial belief in this project and her unwavering support ever since. We would like to thank the entire team at Fair Winds Publishing for bringing this manuscript to life and especially Jill Alexander for sharing our vision of what this book could be.

To a valued friend, Julie Herman, your advice is always brilliant. A special thanks to Brad Herman and Rebecca Beckler for the outstanding photos in this book. We also thank the researchers working to better understand this condition and how to treat it. Our sincere appreciation for those IC patient advocacy groups—particularly the ICA—fighting for IC awareness; patients are fortunate to have such strong support.

Most of all, thank you to all my patients with IC. Your courage, drive, and perseverance are a daily inspiration. I hope that, with this book, I am able to give something back to a group of people who have given me so much.

ABOUT THE AUTHORS

Nicole Cozean, P.T., D.P.T., W.C.S., is one of 275 board-certified pelvic floor physical therapists in the United States and the first physical therapist to serve on the ICA Board of Directors. Her South California clinic, PelvicSanity, specializes in treating pelvic pain conditions in both women and men, including interstitial cystitis. She founded PelvicSanity.com and developed educational courses with the goal of bringing practical, positive information to patients beyond the walls of her own clinic.

Nicole routinely lectures at universities and educates both patients and practitioners across the country through her online courses. In addition to her work in the field of pelvic floor physical therapy, Nicole is the medical director for the East Africa Partnership, overseeing more than forty health care clinics in East Africa. Among other honors, Nicole received Chapman University's Physical Therapy Alumnae of the Year Award.

Jesse Cozean, M.B.A., is a medical researcher and author, and currently serves as the vice president of research and development for the Zylast line of hand sanitizers. He has published peer-reviewed articles in several journals and holds multiple patents in the medical field. Jesse is also the author of *My Grandfather's War: A Young Man's Lessons from the Greatest Generation* (Globe Pequot Press, 2012).

Together, Nicole and Jesse manage PelvicSanity in Laguna Hills and make their home in Orange County, California.

Index

Page numbers in italics refer to illustrations.